T0381478

MEDICAL USES OF MARIJUANA

By: Joseph W. Jacob B.A., M.P.A.

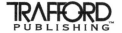
TRAFFORD
PUBLISHING™

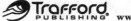 Trafford
PUBLISHING® www.trafford.com

North America & international
toll-free: 1 888 232 4444 (USA & Canada)
phone: 250 383 6864 • fax: 250 383 6804 • email: info@trafford.com

Also Published by:

LIBERTY
PUBLISHING

Canada

TABLE OF CONTENTS

INTRODUCTION

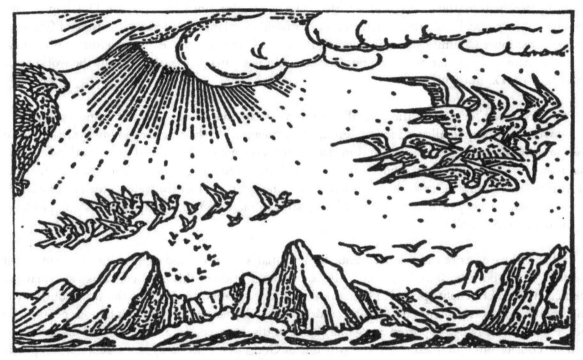

Footnote[1]

Throughout history, God and Mother Nature have provided many valuable medicines that sustain life, relieve pain and promote healing. Aloe vera, for example is a medicinal plant, that for many centuries has relieved pains and helped heal injuries from cuts or burns. Similarly, garlic, onions and apples contain medical properties that help relieve respiratory harms. This book primarily discusses another natural medical resource, the marijuana plant known during the history of mankind to have been successfully used for resolving numerous medical disorders, while also providing many other valuable, practical and constructive uses. In obvious contrast, drinking *alcohol* has produced millions of demonstrable harms including factual and substantiated deaths. Although, the word 'marijuana' has been spelled and popularly pronounced in different ways, its beneficial medical uses and healing effects are well documented, since the beginning of recorded history.

The beginning of recorded history extends back about 10,000 years, and as this book explains marijuana has naturally grown since then in virtually every country on earth. In the process, this versatile and healthful plant has been successful with resolving a significant amount of serious medical disorders. For example, marijuana has been a surprisingly helpful medicine for controlling and relieving leprosy and epilepsy. Natural marijuana plants have also been used to help heal wounds, as well as for medically improving arthritis, rheumatism, asthma, eyesight, high blood pressure, cancers, AIDS, cholera, dysentery, blood-poisoning, appetites and teeth problems. In addition, natural marijuana plants have been medically constructive for improving menstruation processes, labour associated with childbirth, hair loss, and curing alcohol addiction, one of society's most real, factual, widespread, and truthfully harmful menaces.

This book has five chapters. Chapter One describes availability, locations and medical uses of natural green herb marijuana plants from the dawn of creation until about zero A.D. Chapter Two presents more medical and other practical uses of marijuana plants, from about the time of Christ to when Christopher Columbus was discovering America. Chapter Three explains additional medical uses and increased popular public support for natural marijuana plants, throughout the world from about 1500 A.D., until 1923.

Chapter Four focuses on the fear filled fourteen year time frame in North America (1923 to 1937) when relatively small and secretive groups of influential legislators changed important taxation laws prohibiting public cultivation and ingestion of God's medically helpful green herb marijuana plants, while allowing increased public ingestion of harm producing alcohol. Also, for the first time in history God's curative cannabis plants became unjustly placed in the newly created man-made legal criminal category of 'narcotic'. No official justification, or logical explanation was ever provided to the democratic public.

Chapter Five describes additional events, studies, analysis, reports and support for marijuana plant products from about 1940 to the present. The conclusion section of this book contains a summary of medical and other benefits provided by natural marijuana plants, throughout the world during the past approximately ten thousand years of recorded history. Also listed are names of famous people who were recorded as having supported using marijuana, or disapproved of drinking alcohol. Described as well are conclusions and questions about why one of God's most medically beneficial, natural plants was quickly stricken from legal use in democratic North America, and subsequently nearly the rest of the world, with reletively few man-made decisions. Governments for the people and by the people were not publicly evident here. In addition, explanations are presented about how marijuana laws produce demonstrable harms while violating several sections of the Canadian Charter of Rights and Freedoms and the United States Constitution.

God did not prohibit using marijuana in his laws the Ten Commandments. Instead, all plants (and other natural resources) were put on earth for providing life, liberty, comfort, pleasantness, security, happiness and joy for all people. Reliability, hope, goodness, trust and truth are consistent characteristics of God. Is God wrong? Is God not to be trusted?

CHAPTER ONE

IN THE BEGINNING

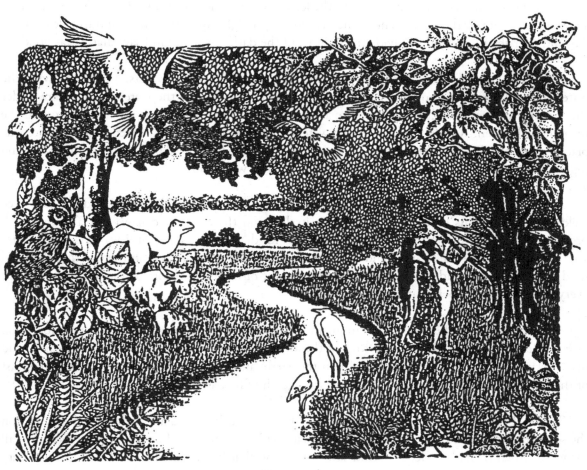

Footnote[2]

By: Joseph W. Jacob B.A., M.P.A.

"IN THE BEGINNING GOD CREATED THE HEAVEN AND THE EARTH. AND THE EARTH was without form and void, and darkness was upon the face of the deep; and the Spirit of God moved upon the face of the waters. And God said: Let there be light, and there was light; and God saw the light, that it was good.

AND GOD DIVIDED the light from the darkness; and God called the light Day, and the darkness he called Night.

AND GOD SAID: Let there be lights in the firmament of the heaven to divide the day from the night; and let them be for signs and for seasons, and for days and for years; and let them be for lights in the firmament of the heaven to give light upon the earth, and it was so. And God made two great lights: the greater light to rule the day, and the lesser light to rule the night. He made the stars also, and God set them in the firmament of the heaven to give light upon the earth, and to rule over the day and over the night, and to divide the light from the darkness, and God saw that it was good.

AND GOD SAID: Let there be a firmament in the midst of the waters, and let it divide the waters from the waters, and God made the firmament, and divided the waters which were under the firmament from the waters which were above the firmament, and it was so; and God called the firmament Heaven. And God said: Let the waters under the heaven be gathered together unto one place, and let the dry land appear, and it was so; and God called the dry land Earth, and the gathering together of the waters called he Seas, and God saw that it was good.

AND GOD SAID: Let the earth bring forth grass, the herb yielding seed and the fruit-tree yielding fruit after his kind, whose seed is in itself, upon the earth, and it was so, and the earth brought forth grass, and herb yielding seed after his kind, and God saw that it was good. . . . These are the generations of the heavens and of the earth when they were created, in the day that the Lord God made the earth and the heavens, and every plant of the field, before it was in the earth, and every herb of the field before it grew.

AND GOD SAID: Let us make Man in our image after our likeness, and let them have dominion over the fish of the sea, and over the fowl of the air, and over the cattle, and over all the earth, and over every creeping thing that creepeth upon the earth; and the Lord God formed man of the dust of the ground, and breathed into his nostrils the breath of life, and man became a living soul. . . .

THUS THE HEAVENS AND THE EARTH were finished, and all the host of them, and on the seventh day God ended his work which he had made, and he rested on the seventh day from all his work which he had made, and God saw everything that he had made, and behold, it was very good. . . .

AND GOD SAID: Behold, I have given you every herb bearing seed which is upon the face of all the earth . . . to you it shall be for meat. . . . I have given every green herb for meat. . . .

AND THE LORD GOD planted a garden eastward in Eden, and there he put the man whom he had formed. . . .

AND THE LORD GOD called unto Adam and said unto him . . . and thou shalt eat the herb of the field . . . till thou return unto the ground, for out of it wast thou taken; for dust thou art and unto dust shall thou return."[3]

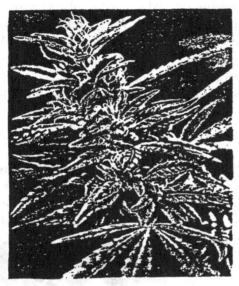

Footnote[4]

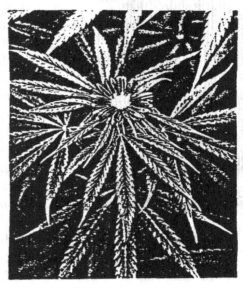

Footnote[5]

Generally speaking, two types of marijuana plants exist: Indica and Sativa. Their leaves, buds, flowers, stocks and resins, also known as: cannabis, marijuana, marihuana, hemp, weed, hash, pot, hashish, nasha, bhang, dagga, ganja, grass, kif, azallu, potamaugus and several other names throughout history are, "an annual herb having angular rough stems and alternate lobed leaves."[6] These plants have been annual herbs throughout the history of mankind. God said, "thou shalt eat the herb of the field."[7] God also said, "I have given every green herb for meat."[8] Because of these directions, God strongly seems to intend that people on earth ingest, eat, or otherwise physically consume his natural green herb marijuana plants. God reinforced this direction of his when he said, "Let us make Man in our image after our likeness, and let them have dominion over all the earth".[9] The word 'all' here is most important.

This direction became reaffirmed as God said, "Behold, I have given you every herb bearing seed which is upon the face of all the earth . . . to you it shall be for meat."[10] As additional reinforcement of his directions, God religiously said, "Let the earth bring forth grass, the herb yielding seed . . . after his kind . . . and God saw that it was good."[11] God would also later direct Moses to use marijuana, as an important ingredient for a special, sacred, holy mixture designed by God to be used by Moses and future generations.[12]

Historical records about human uses of natural green herb marijuana plants also became available from the island of Taiwan, near the southeast corner of China. Archaeologists in this area were

By: Joseph W. Jacob B.A., M.P.A.

successful with unearthing an ancient village, dating back to about 10,000 B.C. Among the ruins were long rod-shaped tools, very similar in design to those later known to have been used for loosening marijuana fibers from their stems.[13] Also found in the same area were pieces of clay-made pottery fragments described as having been decorated, by pressing twisted strands of fibers resembling those of marijuana plants, into their sides while being made. "These simple pots, with their patterns of twisted fibers embedded in their sides suggest that men have been using the marijuana plant in some manner since the dawn of history."[14] Such discoveries demonstrate that many generations of people have constructively used God's natural marijuana plants for at least the last ten thousand years.

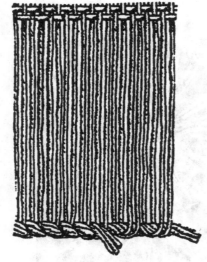

Footnote[15]

Among the first physical human needs to be satisfied by using marijuana plants was the practice of making clothing with it, to provide protection from climatic changes and other environmental hazards. By learning how to weave twisted strands of fibers into clothes, people improved security of their surroundings, not having to rely so much on killing animals for their hides. Ancient Chinese people not only made many clothes with marijuana plants, but they also made sturdy shoes with it.[16]

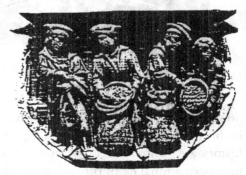

Footnote[17]

Other helpful uses of marijuana plants in ancient China were as important foods and medicines. Vera Rubin concludes, "Besides its importance as a fiber plant, it was also an important food plant, one of the major 'grains' of the ancients.

And, it was an important medicinal plant."[18] Rubin further describes how seeds from marijuana plants were among China's five major grains, along with barley, soybean, rice and millet.[19] Specific descriptions about people legally cultivating and trafficking marijuana plants, "as both a fiber and a grain crop were given in the most ancient works on agriculture in existance."[20]

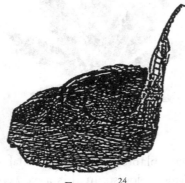

Footnote[24]

Albert Goldman explains other early human uses of marijuana plants were for cooking oils and soap bases.[21] He also describes that marijuana plants grow, "wild all over the world."[22] This supports the moral premise of marijuana plants being put on earth by God, as part of Mother Nature.

Vera Rubin lucidly describes how evidence about people using marijuana was, "found in Neolithic records in northern China."[23] She explains that an archaeologist, Mr. Anderson initially discovered the Neolithic culture in the province of

Honon. It became known as the Yang-shao culture and was similarly characterized by its painted pottery produced about 6,000 years ago. Anderson also believes that traces in the pottery relate to marijuana plants. More archaeological studies subsequently found marijuana plants to be part of Chinese Neolithic cultures, such as the Lung-shan culture of about 4,000 year ago. Additional archaeological records show that marijuana plants have been continuously present in northern China, from at least Neolithic times to the present.[25] Vera Rubin further reveals that fibers from marijuana plants have been used, "since time immemorial for making ropes and fishing nets."[26]

Other important and successful uses of natural marijuana plants in early China were for curative medicines. One ancient humane story is of a Chinese emperor named Liu Chi-nu who had been injured, "and he applied the crushed marijuana leaves to his wound. The medicine healed him, and Liu then announced his discovery to the people of China, and they began using it for their injuries."[27] Another recorded account is of a farmer, who observed a snake placing marijuana on the wound of another snake. The next day it was noticed that the wounded snake was healed. This farmer then, "tested the plant on his own wound and was cured."[28]

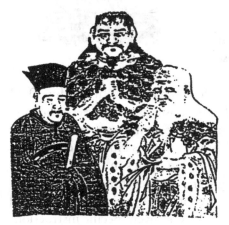

Footnote[30]

A respected and benevolent person, who taught Chinese people about medical uses of marijuana was a famous emperor, Shen-Nung, who lived about 5,000 years ago. He wrote the Pen Ts'ao, an early herbal encyclopedia or standard medical manual as it later became known as. In it marijuana is described as a successful medicine for: "female weakness (menstrual fatigue), gout, rheumatism, malaria, beri-beri, constipation, and absentmindedness."[29] This helpful and humane book (the Pen Ts'ao) became very popular, and its author Shen-Nung was so much liked and respected that he was given, "the singular honor of deification and the title of Father of Chinese Medicine."[31] Shown in the picture are three legendary Chinese emperors: Fu Hei, Shen Nung, and Huang Ti, who became known as respected founders in the art of healing.

A similar description appears in a report to the U.S. Congress, from the Secretary of the U.S. Department of Health, Education and Welfare. This official report explains that medical uses of marijuana are mentioned as early as 2737 B.C., when it was recommended in China for surgical anesthesia, in addition to absentmindedness, constipation, female weakness, and beri-beri.[32]

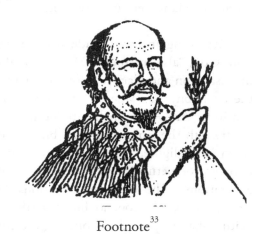

Footnote[33]

This U.S. Government report further describes that marijuana was also medically used in India before 1000 B.C.[34] In India, it has been said many times, those who speak derisively of marijuana, "are doomed to suffer the torments of hell as long as the sun shines in the heavens."[35] According to the Hindu religion in India, "The God Shiva is said to have brought cannabis from the Himalayas for human enjoyment and enlightenment."[36] Enjoyment for *all* people was intended, not merely for a fortunate few. The greatest good for the greatest number became actively and legally practised in many healthful ways.

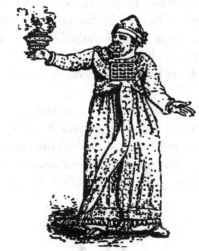

Footnote[40]

Japan is another country regarded similarly to China and India, with its constructive uses of marijuana plants. In Japan, marijuana plants have been used throughout thousands of consecutive years for making helpful items including clothing, bedding, mats and nets. Clothes made from marijuana plants became especially worn at formal or religious ceremonies, because of marijuana's traditional association with purity in Japan.[37] As part of the Shinto religion in Japan, "Cannabis was used for the binding together of married couples to drive away evil spirits and was thought to create laughter and happiness in marriage."[38]

The original Hebrew test of the Old Testament contains references to marijuana plants respectfully used to make incense, "which was an integral part of religious celebration."[39] Marijuana plants also became ingredients for other serious and respected religious ceremonies. In Exodus 30:23 for example, God directs Moses to make a Holy Oil consisting of kanehbosm, myrrh, sweet cinnamon and kassia. Regarding kanehbosm, kaneh was known as marijuana and bosm meant aromatic.[41] God then instructs Moses to anoint the meeting tent and all its furnishings with this Holy Oil containing marijuana plant components by God's design and directions. Anointing things in this way using a 'Holy' Oil containing marijuana was God's method of separating sacred articles from ordinary items. Biblical texts of the Old Testament including Exodus 30:22-33 continue explaining God's good regard for marijuana. Exodus 30:31, for example describes how Moses was given specific instructions by God, "And thou shalt speak unto the children of Israel saying, "This shall be a holy anointing oil unto me throughout your generations."[42] Does this strongly indicate God intends that we use marijuana plants century after century and generation after generation in a continuous manner?

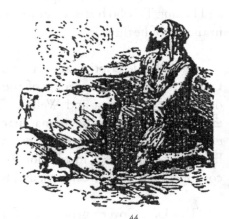

Footnote[44]

Regarding incenses made from marijuana plants, the Lord God, "also instructed Moses to make an altar to burn incense upon and place it before the veil that is by the arc of the testimony . . . where I will meet with thee. The Lord continues: And Aaron shall burn incense every morning when he dresseth the lamps. He shall burn incense upon it. And when Aaron lighteth the lamps at even, he shall burn incense upon it, a perpetual incense before the Lord throughout your generations." The Lord then cautions: "Ye shall offer no strange incense thereon, nor burnt sacrifice, nor meat offering; neither shall ye pour drink offering thereon."[43] Because God seriously approves and encourages people to continuously use marijuana, generation after generation, and we are supposed to approve and support God our superior creator, does it only logically follow that we should approve and support marijuana like God does? Dr. R. Patai, when speaking about historical events expresses the opinion that using sacred oils made partially with marijuana plants, "is based on the belief in its nourishing, conserving and healing powers."[45] Because marijuana is good enough for God, Moses and Aaron, and because God directed Moses to instruct other generations of people about its holy nature, marijuana plants should indeed be good for us, or

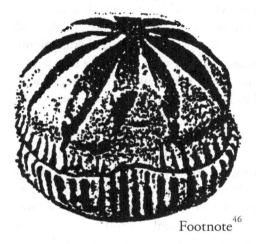

are there those of us who think we can defy God? Some arrogant people perhaps think they are superior to God and contradict his intentions. But disaster and destruction often afflict those who defy God or his directions. Vengeance has many times been said to be within God's domain as in, "Vengeance is mine saith the Lord."

Are our North American man-made laws against people constructively using natural marijuana plants similar to a blasphemous 'slap' in God's face, thinking some mortal people can make an important decision to be superior to that of God's direction? We should often remember, God condemns arrogance and blasphemy. In his original Ten Commandments, the first two are: "I

Footnote [46]

am Yahweh, your God" and, "You shall have no other gods beside me."[47] It should also often be remembered when speaking about mortal people, it was God who said, "for dust thou art and unto dust shalt thou return."[48]

Prohibiting, restricting or denying helpful public uses of medicine from God is most arrogant, because it directly implies that a man-made judgment is superior to God's judgment, which is blasphemous behaviour violating God's first two Commandments. This is partially because mortal people on earth cannot be consistently trusted, whereas God can always be relied on to provide both

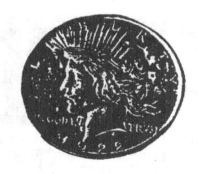

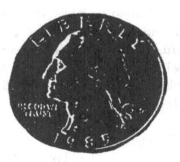

truths and goodness. Many officials in North America have recognized this principle for several decades. Printed distinctively on U.S. currency, along with images of respected leaders including U.S. presidents, such as George Washington are the words, "IN GOD WE TRUST". In essence, when God instructed Moses and Aaron to prepare and use marijuana plant goods, as well as to teach about their goodness, God must be considered to be right because he can always be trusted. Morally, man-made laws against marijuana are hypocritically wrong because they are contrary to God's directions. In Exodus 30:31 God instructs Moses to, "speak unto the children of Israel saying, this shall be a holy anointing oil unto me throughout your generations."[49]

Because God trusts marijuana and we publicly state we trust in God, should we not also trust God's natural marijuana plants to be good for us? When it's good for God, Moses, Aaron, George Washington and Queen Victoria, should it indeed be good for us as well?

Western world laws are typically and historically based on what God has approved, such as his Ten Commandments. So, because God approves of using marijuana as he distinctly does in the Old Testament by instructing Moses to make a special mixture using aromatic marijuana plants (kanehbosm) our laws should approve marijuana as well, because God is supposed to be superior to man, not the other way around. When God directs humanity to use marijuana plants, they indeed should be good for us because as the Bible instructs, "The Lord is my shepard"[50] (not the other way around).

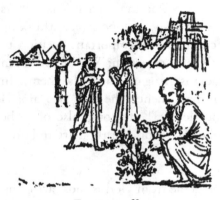

Footnote [52]

Hebrew people had another religious requirement for using marijuana plants, that dead people be buried in kaneh (marijuana) shirts.[51] Are we condemning God and Fathers of the Old Testament, with our modern man-made laws and punishments against people who nonharmfully use marijuana plants? Do you think God, Moses and other sincere leaders of the Old Testament are pleased about it being implied they are fools who don't know what they are talking about? This is what is implied with current world laws that clearly violate and contradict God's directions, instructions and approvals of people using marijuana plants as in the Old Testament. God is never pleased with people who blaspheme against him, and God can mete out most unpleasant punishments.

Even officials from Babylonia, Egypt and Ethiopia enjoyed ingesting healthy marijuana plant goods. "Planno explained that the Great Pyramid at Giza had been built under the direction of an Ethiopian-born pharaoh named Khufu."[53] These leaders liked to smoke the aromatic green herb, "that grew in the valley of Gojam in Ethiopia, the most powerful ganja on the planet, the strain from which Solomon cut a stock which he sowed inside the temple."[54]

Throughout the ancient world Ethiopia was referred to as, "the 'Divine Land' or 'Land of Incense' and was thought to be the home of the gods. The hashish of Ethiopia is generally considered to be superior to that of the Nile Delta. Soil, temperature and humidity make a big difference. Ethiopia played such an important role in history, that it was mentioned as being the Garden of Eden (Genesis 2:12-13)."[55] Another significant use of hashish incenses and special holy anointing oils containing marijuana was for ceremonies involving installation rites of all Hebrew kings and priests. As Doctor R. Patai explains, using this Holy Oil (containing marijuana) is based on humanely providing care to bodies, with its conserving, nourishing

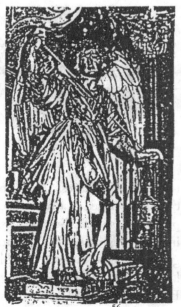

Footnote[56]

and healing powers. He also describes how this custom of anointing kings spread from the ancient Near East to most of Africa.[57] In addition, marijuana and hashish incenses were respectfully used in the temples of Assyria and Babylonia, because the aroma of marijuana smoke became described as being, "pleasing to the gods."[58] This is illustrated in the previous picture with the large swinging incense censer near the floor. It's arrogant, dangerous and foolish for mere mortal people to condemn caring for something that is, "pleasing to the Gods".

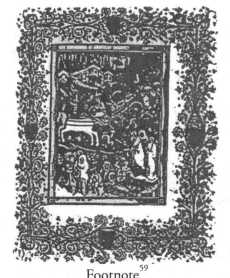

Footnote [59]

The Old Testament also describes how marijuana plants were among the useful merchandise carried by caravans on trade routes of the ancient world. For example, in the original Hebrew of the Bible (Ezekiel 27:19) in a description of Tyre, the 'Royal City' of Phoenicia that became famous for its trade, it is explained that, "Vedon and Yavan traded with yarn for thy wares, massive iron, cassia and kaneh were among thy merchandise."[60] (Again, kaneh was known at the time to mean marijuana plants.) King Solomon, who was a friend of King Hiram of Tyre (960 B.C.) ordered marijuana cords, "for building his temples and throne."[61]

Other prominent developing civilizations also promoted several constructive and respectful uses of God's natural green herb marijuana plants. Vera Rubin and Sula Benet, for example explain that sacred and other beneficial uses of marijuana plants occured in Assyria, Babylonia, Palestine, Scythia and Asia Minor. Herodotus describes Scythian funeral rites involving purification with vapours from marijuana seeds.[62]

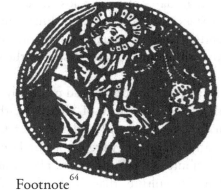

Footnote [64]

In addition Herodotus, "mentions the wild and cultivated hemp of Scythia and describes the hempen garments made by the Thracians as equal to linen in fineness. Hesychius says that Thracian women made sheets of hemp. Moschion (about 200 B.C.) records the use of hempen ropes."[63] Rubin also explains how marijuana plants were used for making the, "ropes of Solomon's temple and robes of the priests."[65] During this time of history near the life of Christ, religious priests who were leaders of church communities respectfully wore and thereby actively approved of using God's green herb marijuana plant products. This was only about two thousand years ago, and the earth was made with God's many green herb plants long before this time.

In addition, God's respectful followers, believers and leaders such as Moses and his children, including priests in religious communities, humanely used and approved of marijuana plants for many practical and respectful purposes. An acknowledged Soviet archaeologist, S.I. Rudenko discovered that Siberian communities in the Altai region constructed burial mounds in which there were bronze vessels containing burned marijuana seeds. "Rudenko believes that these objects were used for funeral purification ceremonies, similar to those practised by the Scythains."[66]

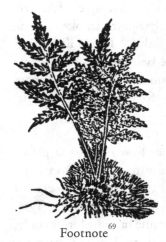

The Atharvaveda, a book written sometime during about 2000 B.C. and 1400 B.C., refers to marijuana as one of the "five kingdoms of herbs . . . which release us from anxiety."[67]

In another historical medical book the Zend-Avesta, the marijuana plant, "occupies first place in a list of 10,000 medicinal plants given to a doctor."[68] People during this time comprehensively studied many of God's plants found in Mother Nature. Of all the different types of plants studied, more than ten thousand became identified and classified as being medically useful plants. And of all these ten thousand various medically beneficial plants, marijuana occupies *first* place on a medical attractiveness list. Much of the impressive Zend-Avesta is, "the teachings of the Persian prophet Zoroaster, who lived around the tenth century, B.C."[70] Both God and objective officials of this time had very positive esteems toward marijuana plants. This feeling also became shared with respected Arabian doctors, during this same period of time, who regarded marijuana as being a useful and, "sacred medicine."[71]

Footnote[69]

Ernest Abel explains that an ancient burial ground was recently unearthed in China. What was found were remnants of the Chou Dynasty, dating from about 1100 B.C. Articles identified in this discovery include pieces of cloth, bronze and jade. Close inspection of the cloth found it to be made of marijuana plant threads, making it the oldest officially known sample of marijuana plants in existence today.[72] Ancient Chinese manuscripts contain numerous passages urging people to plant and cultivate marijuana plants for producing food, medicine, and other beneficial items. A book of ancient Chinese poetry describes the spinning of marijuana threads by a young girl.[73]

Another historical and medically helpful book, the Shu King, written about 2350 B.C., explains that in the province of Shantung, the soil was whitish and rich, laden with resources including marijuana plants, silk and pine trees. Of all these valuable natural resources, marijuana plants were especially honoured as being, "among the articles of tribute."[74] So important a place did marijuana plants occupy in ancient Chinese culture, that the Book of Rites (second century B.C.) describes how, in respect for the dead, mourners wear clothes made from marijuana plants, "a custom followed down to modern times."[75]

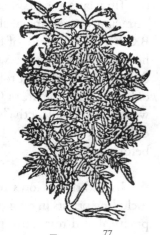

In his book about constructively using marijuana plant products, during the Old Testament, Dr. C. Creighton explains, "Cannabis was the grass eaten by the great Babylonian King Nebuchadnezzar (who ruled from 605 to 652 B.C.) referred to in the Old Testament. . . . Creighton came to the conclusion that the 'grass' which Nebuchadnezzar ate was in fact hashish, or at least some form of cannabis, because the Arabian word for 'grass' was the same as the word for 'cannabis', that is, 'hashish."[76]

Footnote[77]

Physically consuming marijuana became a healthy practise for both royalty and common people.

Even the famous mathematician, Pythagorus received formal recognition for personally consuming marijuana plant goods. "The Book of Lists places Pythagorus (497 B.C.) the Greek philosopher, mathematician and religious reformer first on a list of fifteen people who have taken hashish or marijuana."[78]

Humane uses of God's helpful marijuana plants grew from China to India, and finally to Greece where they became praised as giving comfort to Helen, daughter of Zeus. "It was inevitable that once knowledge of the effects of cannabis became known to the great nations of India and China, it would soon become known to other countries. West of India, in nearby Assyria, scholars became aware of a fascinating plant they referred to in 650 B.C., as Azallu. This plant could not only be used in spinning and in rope-making, but also to dispel depression of the spirit. Cannabis had reached the Middle and Near East, and was so effective that Helen, daughter of Zeus was said to have used it to lull her anguish and sorrow."[79]

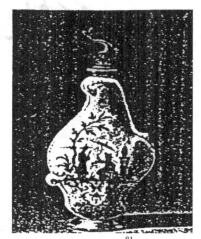

Footnote[81]

Near the end of the nineteen hundreds, an ancient tomb was unearthed near Brandenburg, Germany. Among other things found was a funerary urn dating back to the fifth century B.C. What made this discovery interesting is that the urn, which had been buried in the earth for about 2,500 years contained various identifiable plant fragments, among which were marijuana seeds.[80]

Marijuana plants continued developing as a valuable resource in the Greek Empire. During the third century B.C., Hiero the Second (ruler of the Greek city-state, Syracuse) had his envoys bring back marijuana plants from the Rhone Valley in France, rather than from the Black Sea area, that supplied many other Greek cities.[82] Among their numerous benefits, these marijuana plants were used, "to outfit their ships."[83] It is also recorded that manufacturing French fabrics from marijuana plants, "is almost as ancient."[84]

Throughout this early age of documented history, covering nearly ten thousand consecutive years, God's natural marijuana plants gained popularity as being very useful and healthful, in many regions of the world. Marijuana plants became traditionally related to: healing, helping, purity, pleasantness, hope, strength, trust, security, comfort, nourishment, virility and protection.

From the Chinese people to Moses, Aaron and generations of Israelites, marijuana plants were held in honourable esteem for their many medical, religious and other practical purposes. Used as nutritional foods and healthful medicines for healing diseases and other medical disorders, including beri-beri and wounds, while also providing protective products, such as clothing and shoes, marijuana plants produced a respected history of being a valuable, trusted, constructive, versatile and practical natural public resource.

During this time span, several other nations and countries including: Europe, Russia, Africa, Japan, Greece, Phoenicia, Assyria, Babylonia, India and Arabia also relished marijuana plant goods.

Footnote[85]

CHAPTER TWO

NATURAL GROWTH

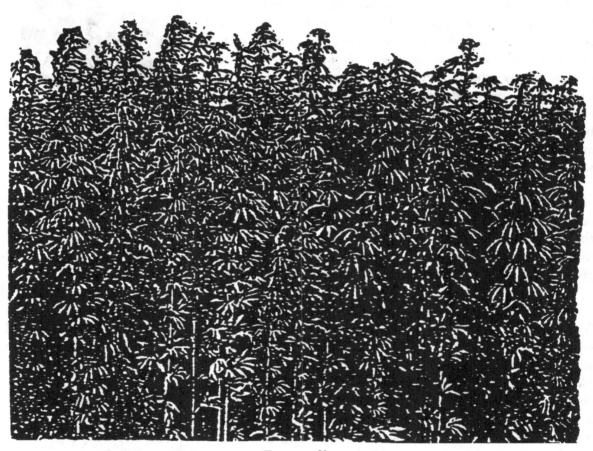

Footnote[86]

This chapter describes additional medical uses of marijuana plants, from about the time of Christ until Christopher Columbus was discovering America. Also explained are other accepted and popular uses of marijuana, and additional areas in the world where marijuana became beneficially used.

During the time of Christ, more prominent medical uses of marijuana plants were for sedative and anesthetic purposes. Dr. R.R. M'Meens, in a report to the Ohio State Medical Society, in 1860 described the impressive use of marijuana plants as a sedative. In support of his view, that this had already been recognized for a long time, he explains how Biblical commentators maintain that the gall and vinegar presented to our Saviour immediately before his crucifixion was, in all likelihood, a preparation of marijuana (hashish) "and even speak of its earlier use."[87] When Christ was born, three Wise Men from the East brought him gifts of gold, frankincense and myrrh. Marijuana plants were known to have been respectfully used for making hashish incenses. Incense "used religiously by the ancient Babylonians was made from cannabis . . . resins collected by hand, from the flowering female cannabis plants. This highly fragrant sticky . . . resin was rolled into balls and short finger-shaped rods, that were traded throughout the ancient world since the remotest times. The ancients called it incense, we call it hashish."[88]

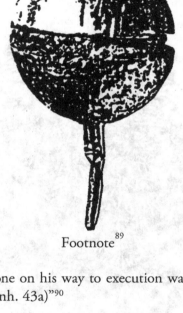

Footnote[89]

Marijuana plant products, such as hashish may well have been responsible for Christ's resurrection, the appearance of dying, with the subsequent appearance of being alive or not dead. In reference to Christ's resurrection, a passage in the Talmud describes, "The one on his way to execution was given a piece of incense in a cup of wine to help him fall asleep. (Sanh. 43a)"[90]

This humane drink was probably called 'Soma' the sacred drink of India at the time. Such a drink, "enabled an adept to enter a deathlike state for several days, and to awaken afterwards in an elated state that lasted a few days more."[91] In addition, the Soma drink likely contained Indian hemp (Cannabis Indica). Marijuana, or Cannabis Indica was, "featured in the drink of Zarathustra.— Holger Kersten, Jesus Lived in India."[92] "If Jesus received a concentrated cannabis extract . . . the resulting cataleptic state induced could easily have been mistaken for death, by his Roman executioners. His limbs would have been stiffening, heartbeat and breathing imperceptible, blood coagulating on his wounds, and flies landing on a still body that resembled a corpse. . . . With Pilate's permission, Joseph removed the body of Jesus from the cross. He was accompanied by Nicodemus. And there also came Nicodemus, who . . . came to Jesus by night, and brought a mixture of myrrh and aloes about a hundred pound weight (John 19:39). One hundred pounds is an enormous amount of the spices to have on hand."[93] After Christ was removed from the cross and placed in a nearby

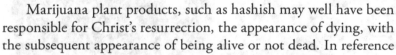

Footnote[94]

tomb, "Nicodemus had laid in a large supply of medicinal herbs, used specifically to heal physical injuries. . . . Crucifixion victims had recovered before."[95]

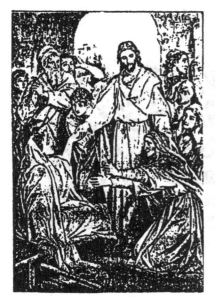

In John's account of the morning of the resurrection, "Mary Magdelene is the first to arrive at the tomb in the garden near the place of execution, where the body of Jesus was lain. She discovered the large stone blocking the tomb's entrance had been rolled away. The gardener addresses her by name, and she then realizes it is Jesus. . . . The face of Jesus was swollen by the injuries."[96]

There is another account of a resurrection in the New Testament. "Lazarus was the man Jesus raised from the dead. (John 12-13). . . . It was after Lazarus's resurrection that many of the Jews "had seen what Jesus did and put their faith in him." (John 11:45)"[97]

It is also recorded, "Jesus gives the disciples an unguent box, and a pouch full of medicine, and tells them to go into the city of habitation and heal the sick. For he says, you must heal the bodies first, before you can heal the heart. Cannabis has been used since ancient times as an unguent (balm for burns and cuts) as the leaves contain a natural antibiotic. Cannabis flowers also have a history as a medicine for countless ills."[99]

Footnote[98]

The hair of Jesus, "is described as flowing and wavy, falling loosely over his shoulders, and was parted in the middle of his head, which was the fashion of the Nazarenes."[100] About, "two years after the crucifixion of Jesus, Paul was on the road to Damascus carrying letters of the high priest of Jerusalem, ordering the synagogues in Damascus to turn over any Nazarenes Paul might find there to be bound for return to Jerusalem. Paul's infamy had preceded him, and Jesus intercepted him outside of Damascus, "saying unto him, "Paul, Paul, why persecutist thou me?" And he said, "Who art thou, Lord?" And the Lord said, "I am Jesus whom thou persecutist. . . . And he trembling and astonished said, "Lord, what wilt thou have me do?" And the Lord said unto him, "Arise and go into the city, and it shall be told there what thou must do." (Acts 9:3-6).[101]

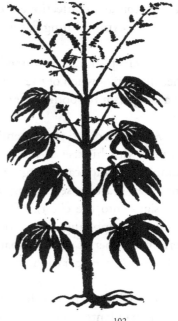

A Sufi/Christian group in Western Afganistan, the followers of Isa, son of Maryam (Jesus son of Mary) claims to have detailed knowledge about the life of Christ after his Crucifixion. In a description from, "Among the Dervishes", O.M. Burke states that he initially assumed the estimated one thousand members of this group were reconverted to Christianity. . . . However, he goes on to state: From their own accounts, and what I could observe, they seem to come from some much older source.

Footnote[102]

According to these people, Jesus escaped from the Cross, was hidden by friends, was helped to flee to India, where he had been before during his youth, and settled in Kashmir, where he is revered as an ancient teacher, Yuz Asaf."[103] Kashmir evolved to become the hashish capital of the world, where multitudes of helpful and healthful marijuana plants freely flourished, without impediments from man-made laws.

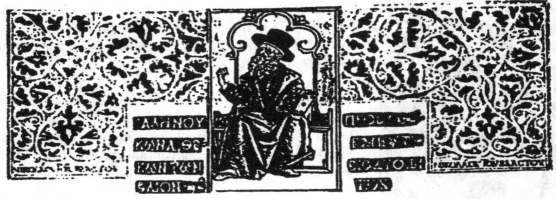

Footnote[104]

Natural marijuana plants grew in popularity providing increasing numbers of people with more healthy foods and medicines. "The classical world offers additional commentary on the use of hemp. Pliny, in the first century A.D., quotes the description of Democritus concerning the use of Potamaugis. . . . This was probably hemp. . . . A few years later, Dioscorides accurately described and illustrated the hemp plant . . . commenting about its use in rope manufacturing, and its curative powers in cases of earache, edema and assorted ills."[105]

About 175 A.D., the famous physician Galen, shown in the previous drawing, "reported the use of cannabis as a confectionery dessert . . . when taken after meals. . . . He humanely recommended its use for extinguishing flatus, curing earache and other problems."[106]

When speaking about medical uses of marijuana, respected Dioscorides, who was described as the, "most renowned of the ancient writers on material medica, recommended the seeds, in the form of a cataplasm to soothe inflammation."[107]

A respected and well-intentioned Chinese surgeon, Hua T'o, in the second century A.D. became famous with his use of marijuana plants for anesthetic purposes. He is said to have successfully completed complicated surgery, "without causing pain. Among the amazing operations he performed are organ grafts, resectioning of intestines, laparotomies (incisions into the loin) and thoractomies (incisions into the chest)."[108] All of these very complex surgical operations were said to be made painless by applying an anesthetic prepared with using marijuana resin as an ingredient. "After a certain number of days, the patient finds he has recovered, without having experienced the slightest pain during the operation."[109]

The Chinese people humanely used many parts of marijuana plants for medicines. Tops of marijuana plants, including flowers are medically recommended for 120 different forms of diseases. "The seed coat and its adhering resin were used to stimulate the nervous system, the seeds themselves were used to counteract inflammations and skin irritations, and are considered tonic (mentally or morally invigorating) a restorative of good health, laxative, diuretic, and excellent for worming babies and animals. The oil was used as a hair tonic, and to counteract sulphur poisoning, the fresh juice of the leaves was used for treating scorpion bites."[110] In addition, tops of flowering marijuana plants, "were frequently recommended for constipation, difficult childbirth, menstrual cramps, rheumatism, convulsions and fevers."[111]

Another practical use of marijuana plants, during this time was making good quality paper with it. In China, near the end of the Han dynasty, a Marquis named Ts'ai Lun prepared a mixture of old fish nets, rags, marijuana fibers and wooden bark. The finished product was paper, which he presented to the country's royal throne in 105 A.D. (Fish nets had often been made with marijuana plants.)[112] However, the oldest known existing paper made with marijuana plant components was recently discovered in a grave, from the Shensi province of China. It dates to before the reign of Emperor Wu, of the Early Han dynasty, at about the time Christ lived.[113]

By 500 A.D., royalty in France also enjoyed ingesting marijuana plant products. Here, marijuana received special attention involving burial ceremonies for the deceased. The tomb of France's Queen Arnegunde, who was buried in Paris around 570 A.D. contained gold coins, expensive jewelry, rich garments and marijuana. These earthly treasures were all encouraging expressions, with the intention of the deceased person to enjoy, "as comfortable a life in the next world, as that from which their soul had just departed."[114]

Another region of the world where marijuana grew more popular was in Tibet. Here, during the seventh century A.D., marijuana plants became an important part of the Tantric religion. The Dali Lama ('mighty superior') and other priests of the religion called Lamas ('superiors') consumed marijuana plants, "to overcome evil forces."[116]

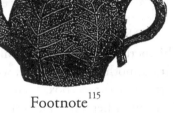

Footnote[115]

By about three hundred years later, Chinese doctors had discovered other valuable medical uses of marijuana. Drinking teas, eating seeds and smoking resins and leaves from marijuana plants produced pleasant results for reducing and eliminating medical disorders and discomforts. Notice how the broad leaves designed on the previous tea pot are very similar to healthy leaves from marijuana 'Indica' plants. Also, a close look shows it's handle resembles the stock of a wholesome marijuana plant. Long narrow leaves designed on the outside of the tea pot below resemble those of marijuana 'Sativa' plants. This type of plant was primarily native to Europe and North America, whereas marijuana Indica plants flourished more predominantly in Asia.

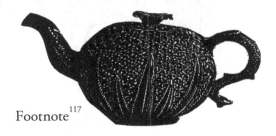

Footnote[117]

T'ang Shen-wei, during the tenth century humanely explains that marijuana products were beneficial for healing waste diseases and injuries, as well as for clearing blood, cooling body temperatures and relieving fluxes (such as high blood pressure) in addition to helping with curing rheumatism, and promoting the discharge of pus.[118] Physical improvements from such medical disorders naturally produced better health conditions and longer life expectancies for those who actively participated.

"About 950 A.D., an Arabian physician noted that the hemp that was used for rope-making could ease headaches."[119] Marijuana helped reduce physical and mental medical disorders. Aboriginal Indians in North America also respectfully used natural marijuana plants. The Hemp Museum in Amsterdam reports, "stone and wooden pipes and hemp fiber pouches were found in the Ohio Valley from about 800 A.D."[120] Pipes and chellums for smoking marijuana leaves, tops and resins were also being made and used in Africa, Asia and Europe at this time.

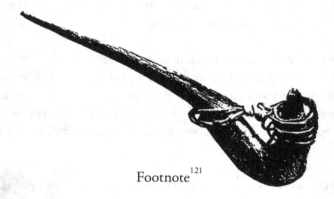

Footnote[121]

A Native American Indian from California named Rainbow Speaks, religiously explains, "smoking this herb is a prayer of thanksgiving to the Great Mother. Rainbow, age seventy-nine recalls his Grandmother's daily ritual, when he was a small child. She took some cannabis flower tops out of an intricately carved box, then rolled it in handmade corn paper. She held the resulting 'joint' upright in front of her, and watching the rising, swirling smoke prayed: "Oh thank-you Great Mother!" To this day, Native Americans continue lifting pipes filled with the sacred herb, in offerings of thanks to the Great Mother."[122]

North American aboriginal Indians learned and appreciated benefits from using marijuana plants, as with traditional 'peace pipes'. "Long before other nations came to this continent, native peoples had knowledge of this sacred plant, this sacred medicine.

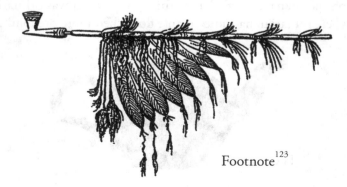

Footnote[123]

We understood that it could help one breathe better, it could help one see better, it could help one attune themselves to the harmonies . . . of Creation. When one smoked the natural plants, one came closer to the natural powers of creation."[124]

India is another country where people continued developing more medical uses of marijuana. By the end of the 10th century, marijuana received praise there as being, "the food of the gods."[125] Soon thereafter, records from India medically describe marijuana as being, "joyful."[126] Other related medical uses of ingesting marijuana include: astringency (a reduction in the size of a body canal) for reducing excessive discharge (such as in stopping a nose bleed); the ability to help remove unwanted wind and phlegm, as well as its ability to improve personal speaking, mental development and bodily heat.[127] More medical uses of marijuana in India involve providing people with additional energy, "to arouse appetite and as . . . a source of great staying-power under severe . . . fatigue."[128] Staying power requires energy for both mental and physical persistence, perserverance, continuous alertness and successful completions.

Mark David Merlin explains how footmen from India, who packed goods up the Himalayan mountains ingested marijuana products for obtaining additional energy. Marijuana plant goods also became useful for, "effectively removing dandruff and vermin from hair, reducing pain from earaches, alleviating bowel complaints, such as diarrhea and constipation, and checking discharge from gonorrhea. Other medical uses of marijuana recorded in India include relieving: headaches,

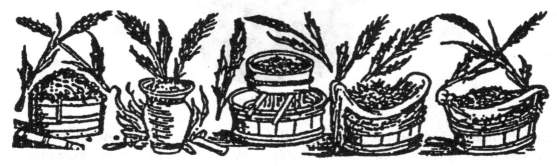

Footnote[129]

acute mania, whooping cough, asthma and insomnia."[130]

When describing benefits from physically ingesting marijuana plant buds, leaves and resins, the humane Persian leader Haydar, about 1150 A.D. told his followers, "God has granted you the

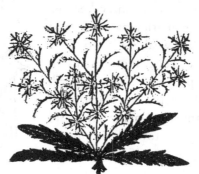

Footnote[131]

privilege of knowing the secret of these leaves. Thus, when you eat it, your dense worries may disappear, and your exalted minds may be come polished."[132] Joy increases.

A famous Benedictine Monk and qualified Bachelor of Medicine at this time, Francois Rabelais was so favourably impressed with using marijuana plants, that in his estimation, they stood at the very pinnacle of plant life. With these plants, I have, "found so much efficacy and energy, so much completeness and excellency, so much exquisiteness and rarity, and so many admirable effects."[133]

During the late 1400s, France continued enthusiastically developing and increasing uses of marijuana plants. Legal planting, cultivating, buying, selling, using, trading, importing, exporting, transporting and trafficking all lawfully developed a trend of expansion and prosperity. "This most prosperous kingdom, declared the Chancellor of France in 1484 has a great number of provinces, which because of the beauty of the countryside, the fertility of the

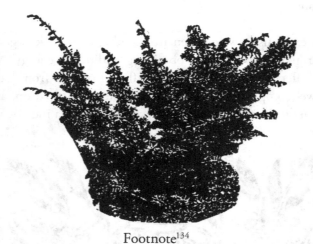

Footnote[134]

soil, and the health-giving air easily surpasses all the countries on earth."[135] At this time, French farmers were regularly encouraged to work very diligently, in producing better and more amounts of wool, flax and especially marijuana plants.[136]

France also developed as an attractive international producer and exporter of multi-useful marijuana plants, during the 1400s and 1500s. So respected and popular were France's commercial products, that this country became known as having two major exports: marijuana plants and wheat, enthusiastically attracting, "the wealth of Europe."[137] France was soon selling to England alone, more than two million pounds of marijuana plants per year.[138] Many typical, moral, productive and respected people were naturally consuming marijuana, without any man-made laws and punishments impeding their progress towards improved health and wealth.

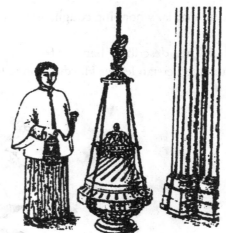

Footnote[139]

Even the Catholic Bible doesn't discourage people from consuming marijuana. "God makes the earth yield healing herbs, which the prudent man should not neglect. Sirach: 38:4 (Catholic Bible)"[140] Other respected Biblical commentators conclude, "We find that the use of cannabis is never forbidden or even discouraged in the Bible. Some passages directly refer to the goodness of using herbs like cannabis."[141]

Christian clergy regularly ate and otherwise consumed marijuana plant components. "Monks were required to eat hemp seed dishes three times a day, to weave their clothes of it, and to print their Bibles on paper made with its fiber."[142]

Ground-up marijuana seeds were also eaten as a nutritious and delicious butter. "Hemp seed can be ground into a paste, similar to peanut butter only more delicate in flavor."[143] Udo Erasmus, (Ph.D.) nutritionist explains how marijuana plant seed, "butter puts our peanut butter to shame for nutritional value. The ground seeds can be baked into breads, cakes and casseroles."[144] In the olden days, peasants ate hemp seeds and were more resistant to disease.[145] Should this tell us something? Should we be learning from history to improve the future? Being more resistent to disease is

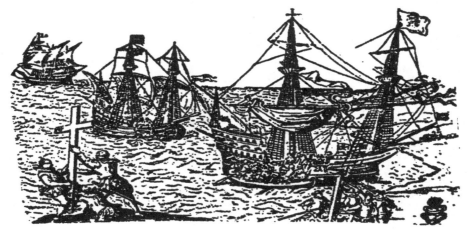

Footnote[146]

medically beneficial for people who want to live longer healthier lives, with less pains, miseries, medical harms, restrictions and costs.

During this second time range of nearly fifteen hundred years, from about the time of Christ to when Columbus was discovering America, many additional valuable and healthful uses grew from marijuana buds, leaves, resins, stocks, flowers, roots and seeds. They became successfully useful as sedatives and anesthetics. They were also physically consumed for healing: waste diseases, injuries, rheumatism, and respiratory problems, including, asthma and whooping cough. Marijuana also became medically useful for helping to clear blood in bodies, and for reducing high blood pressure. In addition, marijuana provided healthful physical and mental energies to human bodies. During this time, marijuana also became seriously and respectfully used for sacred religious purposes, including purification efforts to expel evil forces, in addition to intending future comforts for deceased persons.

By: Joseph W. Jacob B.A., M.P.A.

Other respectful and constructive uses of marijuana plants included: making robes for priests, food for clergy, with laughter and happiness in marriage.

Foods, clothes, medicines, shelters, oils, sails, ropes, nets and papers resulted as practical products made from marijuana plants. Many of these marijuana-plant-made goods were likely aboard the Santa Maria, as Columbus discovered America.

CHAPTER THREE

MORE HEALTHY MEDICINE

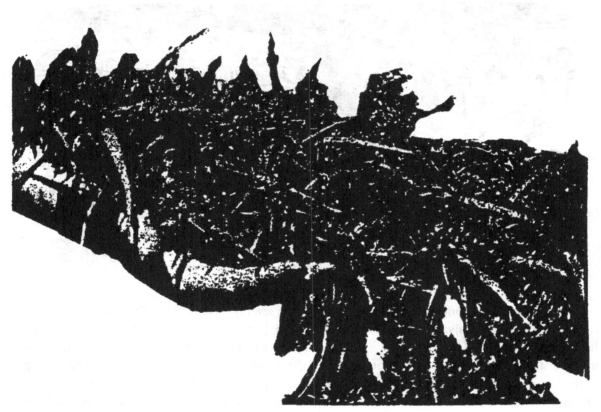

Footnote[147]

By: Joseph W. Jacob B.A., M.P.A.

This chapter explains more medical and other practical uses of marijuana, from when Columbus was discovering America to the beginning of alcohol prohibition and untrue published stories against God's green herb cannabis plants during the early 1920s. Also listed are several prominent people, who have actively encouraged using marijuana, or denounced drinking alcohol. Some such famous people include: President George Washington, Queen Victoria, Queen Elizabeth the First, King James the First, Samuel de Champlain (Father of Canada), President John Adams, President Thomas Jefferson and Benjamin Franklin. Many countries who legally encouraged commercial and public cultivation, processing and beneficial uses of marijuana, during this third time-span include: China, India, Africa, Arabia, England, France, Russia, Germany, Spain, Italy, Ireland, Holland, Poland, Sweden, Czechoslovakia, Argentina, Switzerland, the United States and Canada.

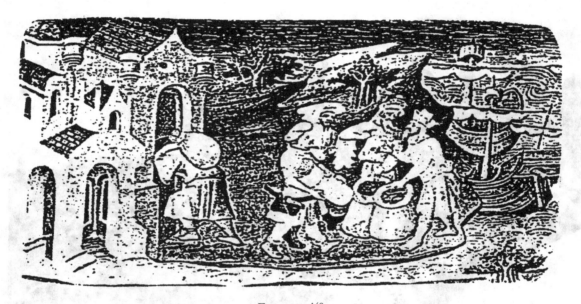

Footnote[148]

India, like China continued humanely developing several successful medical uses of marijuana. A book named the Rajvallhaba, written about medical benefits describes marijuana as follows. It, "destroys leprosy. It creates vital energy, increases mental powers and internal heat, corrects irregularities of the phlegmatic humor, and is an elixir vitae."[149] For joy, it is used, "to bring delight to the kings of gods (Siva) it was called vijaya (victorious) . . . believed to have been obtained by men on earth for the welfare of all people."[150] Complimenting God's instructions to Moses, people in Asia also respectfully regarded marijuana as being humanely beneficial for the welfare of all people, not merely for a fortunate few. Eliminating discrimination, along with improving life, liberty, health, security, protection and personal comfort levels for everyone, became a sincere concern of these humane leaders.

Marijuana also received usefulness for spiritually purifying peoples' behaviours. When physically consumed in the early morning marijuana, "is believed to cleanse the body of sin"[151] (as well as congestion). In India, where marijuana is called bhang, it became seriously and religiously believed, "No good thing can come to the man who treads underfoot the holy bhang leaf."[152] Here again, much respect was regularly practiced and encouraged for marijuana. In Asia, a pleasant expression advises that a longing or yearning for marijuana, "foretells happiness."[153] Very positive, respectful and optimistic characteristics grew with green herb marijuana plants.

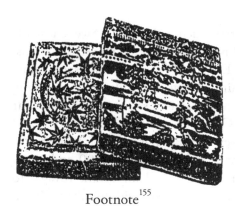

Footnote[155]

Other humane medical uses of marijuana in India are recorded as being successful cures for: fevers, dysentery and sunstroke, as well as for: clearing phlegm, quickening digestion, sharpening appetites, making clear the speech of lispers, freshening intellects, and giving alertness to people.[154] Marijuana and hashish also received a description of being: a solace in discomfort, a cure in sickness, and a guardian whose gracious protection saves people from attacks of harmful evil influences.[156] Because of these many medical and spiritual attributes, marijuana became related to: calming, healing, hope, comfort, trust, security, joy and respect.

In Russia, Poland and Lithuania, marijuana became medically useful for reliving tooth aches. A dental practioner named Szyman, during the 1500s prescribed the following procedure for removing unwanted organisms from teeth. After boiling water in a new pot, marijuana seeds and heated rocks are added. When resulting vapours are inhaled, it causes unwanted organisms to leave peoples' teeth.[157] Not only were medical uses of marijuana increasing in Asia at this time, but demands for marijuana plant products continued significantly increasing throughout Europe. In England, around 1533 for example, King Henry the Eighth commanded: for every sixty acres of farmland a person owned, a quarter of an acre was to be planted, or sown with marijuana seeds.[158] The penalty for *not* doing this was, "three shillings and four pence."[159] Demands for marijuana plants kept rapidly growing.

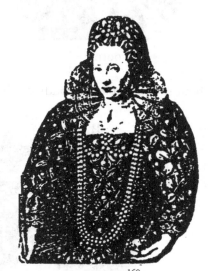

Footnote[160]

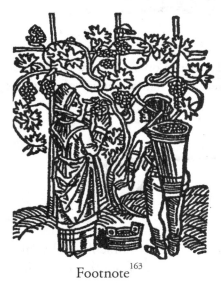

Footnote[163]

Thirty years later, his loyal daughter Queen Elizabeth I reissued this official order, but raised the penalty to five shillings.[161] At the same time, many additional beneficial uses were being humanely developed with marijuana plants, in day-to-day life styles of people throughout Great Britain. Productive public participants from England, Ireland, Wales and Scotland eagerly supported Queen Elizabeth I and her requirement for legally growing and cultivating millions of marijuana plants. Multipurpose marijuana plants were very useful in England for making: ship and windmill sails, ropes, bags, blankets, sheets, caulking, paints, oils, fine napkins, flags and altar cloths.[162]

As civilization progressed, other major countries and nations encouraged development and more uses of natural marijuana plants. France was buying large quantities of

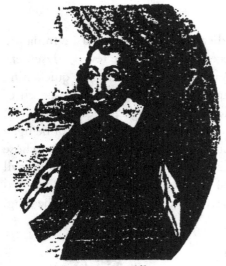

Footnote[165]

marijuana from countries such as Italy and Sweden, while selling vast volumes of marijuana to other powerful nations, including Spain and England.[164] During this same time, Canada and its governing officials had difficulties obtaining sufficient quantities of marijuana for satisfying local popular demands. Samuel de Chaplain, a courageous explorer and 'Father of Canada' (New France) was a practical supporter of cultivating marijuana plants. Between 1600 and 1605, Samuel de Champlain made several important voyages to Canada, and brought marijuana seeds with him.[166] By 1606, marijuana plants were, "growing in Port Royal, in Nova Scotia, under the watchful eye of the colony's botanist and apothecary, Louis Hebert."[167] In 1610, Louis Hebert brought his wife to Canada, "marking the first time that a white woman had set foot in the new world."[168] In the picture below, Louis Hebert talks with a Micmac Indian, likely about marijuana leaves, buds, seeds and resins.

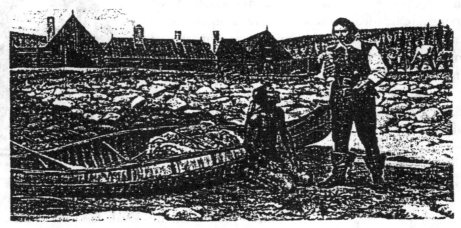

Footnote[169]

Shown below is a Micmac Indian smoking pipe, used when Louis Hebert, Samuel de Champlain and other Europeans were settling in Canada, where they had a scarcity of cannabis

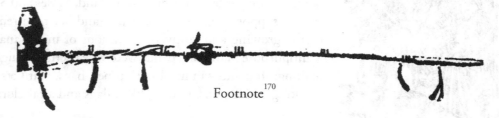

Footnote[170]

(marijuana) plants. Jean Talon, Canada's first Finance Minister had so much difficulties obtaining sufficient amounts of green herb marijuana plants, that he legally confiscated from the inhabitants, all of the available sewing thread in Quebec, announcing he would sell it back only in return for marijuana plants.[171] This immediately encouraged many responsible housewives to be eagerly involved with planting, cultivating, harvesting, transporting, trafficking and selling marijuana, for sewing thread, so vitally needed when making family clothing. Here, only Jean Talon and his appointed designates could legally issue sewing thread, in return for marijuana plants, during this difficult scarcity of helpful cannabis goods. Canadian Finance Minister Talon also gave many marijuana seeds, "free to farmers, with the understanding, that they were to plant

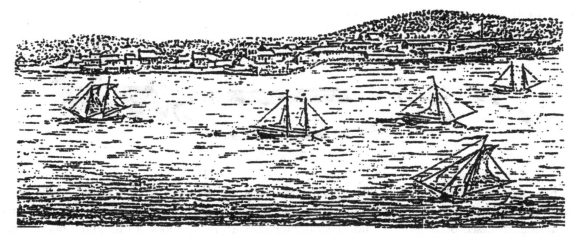

Footnote[172]

them immediately and replace the gift with seeds from their next year's crop."[173] In 1763, Canada's Governor of Quebec was told *not* to grant any land to any settler, unless he was willing to cultivate marijuana plants on it.[174]

In 1790, Canadian governmental officials co-ordinated transportation and delivery, of two thousand bushels of marijuana seeds, from Russia to Quebec, that were then distributed free of charge to all agricultural districts in the province.[175] Governing parliaments of Canada also implemented additional methods for legally encouraging large-scale planting, cultivating, transporting, buying, selling and trafficking of marijuana plants in Canada. For example, near the beginning of the 1800s, Parliament made an offer to James Campbell and another farmer Charles Grece, both of whom were experts in cultivating and processing marijuana plants in Europe. If either of them were to plant or sow twenty-five acres of land, with marijuana seeds during their first year of settlement in Canada, and agree to continue cultivating marijuana plants at a rate acceptable to local authorities after that, and if they were willing to teach settlers how to effectively grow marijuana plants, and be inspectors of marijuana plants produced, they could expect to receive the following benefits. First they would be assured a substantial purchase price of forty-three pounds per ton, for all marijuana plants produced, for five years. (This was known to be a very attractive amount of money at the time.) In addition, each of these men would be paid two hundred pounds per year, as well as be given a loan of four hundred pounds, free passage to Canada, one hundred and fifty acres of land, free marijuana seeds, and money for paying marijuana 'dressers'. The governing Parliament of Canada also promised to pay each of these agricultural gentlemen a lifetime annuity of two hundred pounds, if this venture became successful.[176]

Additional subsequent promises of seventy pounds per ton and three hundred acres of land were made to any person who cultivated and harvested five tons of marijuana plants during a single year in Canada. "To make sure these offers were heard throughout the country, they were issued from church pulpits, immediately after church services were concluded."[177] Because of the great demand for these helpful and versatile plants, large and small scale cultivations of marijuana crops flourished, with continuous legal approval in Canada, from thousands of years before the 1600s, until 1923. Marijuana production efforts were traditionally encouraged by effective, respected and humane Canadian leaders, improving lives for the people.

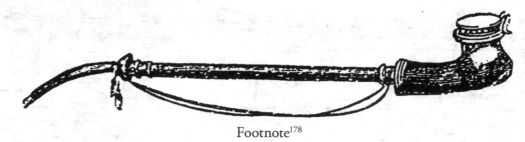

Footnote[178]

In Arabia during this time, doctors praised marijuana as being a helpful sacred medicine. A person named Syrenius explained that marijuana became successfully useful, as a remedy for burns. In addition, diseased body joints could be straightened, with using roots of marijuana plants, that had been boiled in water.[179] Beneficial medical uses of marijuana continued increasing, leading to improved health standards for involved free choice participants.

Free countries of the United States and England, also experienced shortages of marijuana, similar to the scarcity situation in Canada. During the reign of Queen Elizabeth I, for example, supplies of marijuana plants could not keep up with strong demands in England. This was partially because of Britain's expanded naval fleet, which seriously relied on using oodles of marijuana plants.[180]

Inferior substsitutional options, such as domestic flax, for example, had short strands of fibers, that were not as suitable as marijuana, for making sails and ropes. To compound the British naval fleet's supply shortage of marijuana, a trade conflict developed between England and Holland, whose ships were supplying England with marijuana plants, that were grown in the Baltics and areas of the Dutch East Indies. This conflict caused an acute shortage of marijuana, not only in England, but in the United States as well.[181]

Another international effort, for increasing supplies of marijuana occurred in 1611, when the first officially known crops of marijuana Indica seeds, from India were planted, in the United States near Jamestown, Virginia.[182] Early settlers in the United States were also officially encouraged to plant, cultivate and harvest marijuana plants. The Pilgrims, for example, who landed at Plymouth Rock, in 1620 came to America, because they were assured, "they could practice their religious beliefs in freedom."[183] With serious religious fervor and respect, marijuana plants became one of the first crops grown, in this new Massachusetts colony.[184] The General Court of Massachusetts, also officially encouraged new colonists to grow marijuana plants, so durable clothes could be made with them, among many other helpful items. This Court concluded, that the new colony could freeze to death during the winter, and as a result, it directed all masters of families in the colony to have their children and servants spend more time cultivating marijuana plants.[185] For countless continuous years, children in China, India, Asia and Europe traditionally participated in cultivating and consuming marijuana plants. No related marijuana-produced harms ever became factually recorded and truthfully substantiated.

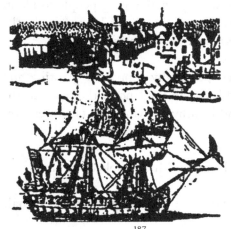

Footnote[187]

In 1629, ship building began in the new village of Salem, Massachusetts. However, builders, owners and merchants could not obtain sufficient quantities of marijuana plants to properly outfit their new ships. Marijuana, "was so scarce, that it had to be imported from abroad."[186] Shortly after this, the Massachusetts Court passed a law requiring every householder to plant marijuana seeds.[188]

King James I of England, also ordered settlers in the United States to produce marijuana plants, as well as iron, flax and silkgrass.[189] Marijuana plants grown in American became, "excellent for bagging, webbing, twine and marine rope."[190] It is recorded by 1630, half the winter clothes and nearly all of the summer clothes in America were made from marijuana plants.[191]

In 1640, the General Assembly of Connecticut encouraged its colonists to grow marijuana plants so, "we might, in time have a supply of linen cloth among ourselves."[192] Here too, the General Assembly feared colonists would die from exposure, if they didn't grow marijuana plants for making their clothes with.[193]

Another large country continually trying to plant, cultivate and harvest more marijuana during this time was Russia. Cities like Saint Petersburg and Riga became international export centers for Russian marijuana.[194] Russia progressively developed as one of the few international trading countries in the world, where there was more marijuana plants being cultivated and harvested than was being locally consumed. By 1630 for example, Russia was supplying greater than ninety percent of London's marijuana demands, and by 1633 this volume continued increasing to about ninety-seven percent.[195]

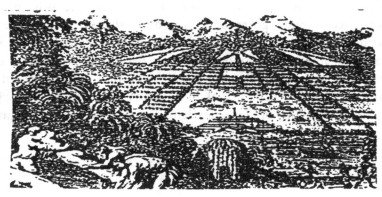

Footnote[196]

By: Joseph W. Jacob B.A., M.P.A.

Throughout the U.S., farmers continued cultivating hemp (marijuana) plants, contending with difficult growing conditions, fluctuating prices and superior quality Russian marijuana.[197] However, both federal and state governments in the U.S. kept enthusiastically encouraging people to plant, cultivate, harvest, process, transport, traffic and consume marijuana plants. In 1762 for example, the state of Virginia imposed punishments against those who did *not* cultivate marijuana plants.[198]

George Washington, first President of the United States, personally supported planting and cultivating marijuana (hemp). President Washington enjoyed living in the land of the free and the home of the brave. He encouraged nonharmful freedoms and healthy growing results. An excerpt from his diary describes the following.

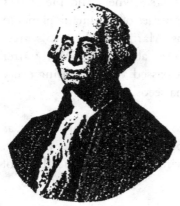

Footnote[200]

"1765 May 12-13 Sowed Hemp at Muddy hole by swamp.

August 7 began to separate . . . the Male from the Female hemp . . . rather too late."[199]

As previously explained, hemp plants and marijuana plants are the same as cannabis plants. Experienced growers and processors knew that female marijuana plants develop more enhanced medical qualities, if they become separated from male plants before fertilization occurs. The previous phrase, "rather too late" strongly suggests that President George Washington cultivated marijuana plants for their medical values, among other constructive and humane purposes.[201]

In England during this time, many medical uses of marijuana received acknowlegement by the general public. In 1682 for example, the New London Dispensatory wrote that marijuana seeds were being used for curing coughs and jaundice.[202] Oil from the seeds constitute a significant nutritional component.

The New English Dispensatory published in 1764 recommends boiling marijuana plant roots and applying them to the skin, so as to reduce inflammation. Other medical uses of this marijuana-plant-root medicine were for, "drying up tumors and dissolving deposits in the joints."[203] Public medical uses of marijuana continued increasing as time progressed.

England and the United States also successfully used marijuana plants for making paper, upon which money, military commands, government records, business accounts and other important information was written. Around 1675, an English papermaker Mr. Jacob Christian Shaffer wrote an instructional textbook, about the art of papermaking. Because there was an extreme shortage of usual ingredients for making paper, such as linen and rags, Mr. Shaffer suggested using marijuana plant fibers, similar to the Chinese approach of about 105 A.D. To illustrate this idea, Mr. Shaffer printed sections of the third volume of his textbook, on paper made from marijuana plants.[204]

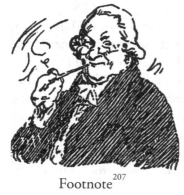

Another trusted and respected pioneer leader, "Benjamin Franklin started one of America's first paper mills with cannabis."[205] It soon became known that paper made from marijuana plants, "lasted 50 to 100 times longer than most preparations of papyrus, and was a hundred times easier and cheaper to make."[206]

In 1777, another American printer Robert Bell who addressed his workshop as, "Next Door to Saint Paul's Church, Third Street, Philadelphia" recommended new paper be made using marijuana plants as a primary natural resource ingredient. He explained, since the United States had declared its independence from England, they could no longer rely on flax or cotton imports.[208]

Footnote[207]

In Virginia at this time, a well-known and respected gentleman, Robert "King" Carter owned more than three hundred thousand acres of farmland, on which he grew and cultivated marijuana plants. He was an, "ancestor of President Jimmy Carter."[209] In 1775 and 1776, this three hundred thousand acre plantation did not grow enough marijuana plants to satisfy public demands. For example, "In 1775, he bought an additional five hundred pounds from his stepbrother. In 1776, he bought two tons more."[210] Among other things, marijuana plants in the United States were being made into 'osnaburg' a coarse clothing fabric used in making shirts and trousers for soldiers and workers.[211]

Shortly after the beginning of the American Revolution in 1775, the U.S. Congress officially requested colonists to cultivate as many marijuana plants as possible. A serious and practical U.S. Congressional intention here, among other things was to have American colonists make clothing from these marijuana plants. They might then save their lives and those of American soldiers, particularly during the long, frigid, snowy and windy winters.[212] "Had it not been for organizations like the Daughters of Liberty, whose enthusiasm and efforts encouraged

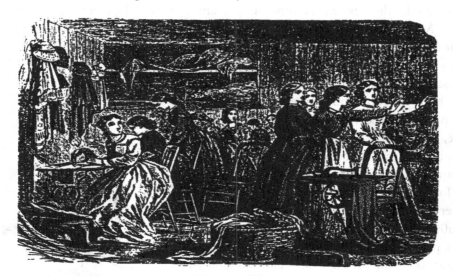

Footnote[213]

colonial women to make their own clothes, the disastrous winter of 1778 at Valley Forge might have been typical of life throughout the northern colonies."[214]

By: Joseph W. Jacob B.A., M.P.A.

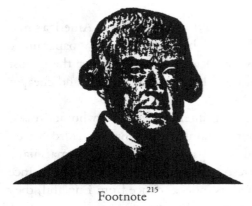

Footnote[215]

Thomas Jefferson, another respected U.S. President also approved of using marijuana plants. In 1781, it became acknowledged that Thomas Jefferson reserved marijuana, "in the back country . . . to be used in paying for articles bought in Philadelphia, for use of the Army."[216] In addition, "Thomas Jefferson wrote and acted on behalf of hemp many times."[217] President Jefferson seriously concluded, "Hemp is of the first necessity to wealth and protection of the country."[218] It is also recorded that President Thomas Jefferson obtained, "rare hemp seeds from Europe for American farmers."[219]

In many places throughout North America, marijuana actually became more valuable than cash during these times. "Cannabis (hemp) was legal tender (money) in most of the Americas, from 1631 until the early 1800s."[220] In addition, people could pay their taxes with marijuana, "throughout America for over 200 years."[221] Paper money often had little value in the colonies. "A thousand dollars in Virginia currency, for example was only worth one dollar in silver. Because of the lack of faith in paper money, the American economy operated on the barter system."[222] And because of marijuana plants', "comparative uniformity and its comparative freedom from deterioration, the universal and steady demand for it, and its value which exceeded all other raw produce, it was recognized as the standard commodity for the first three or four decades of the new American republic."[223]

With Canada, near the end of the American Revolution (1776) governing officials doubled their efforts, for encouraging increased public participation in cultivating more marijuana plants. A public relations campaign was started, announcing marijuana plants were, "a valuable economic commodity to colony and mother country alike."[224] It was logically and economically explained, if production of marijuana increased, "there would be more money and more employment. The standard of living would rise."[225] Marijuana grew freely, with a reliable reputation of humanely improving health, security, protection, peace, prosperity, happiness, joy and uniformity.

When describing major industries of the 1700s and 1800s, it is factually recorded that marijuana, "is, as it has been for thousands of years, the biggest business and most important industry on the planet."[226] At this time, marijuana also progressed into being, "Russia's number one trading commodity—ahead of its furs, timber and iron."[227] When speaking about Russian marijuana, "John Quincy Adams (later U.S. president) who was American Consul at St. Petersburg, 1809 noted as many as 600 clipper ships flying the American flag, in a two week period were in St. Petersburg . . . loading principally cannabis hemp for England . . . and America, where quality hemp is also in great demand."[228] Comparative uniformity and universal demand became two prominent features of valuable and versatile green herb marijuana plants.

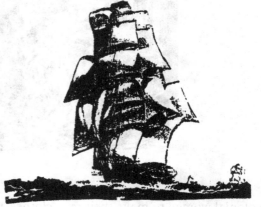

Footnote[229]

In England at this time, further attention focused on increasing medical uses of marijuana. The Edinburgh New Dispensary (1794) as well as prominent medical people of the general area and time reported additional medical benefits from using marijuana, especially with respiratory disorders.

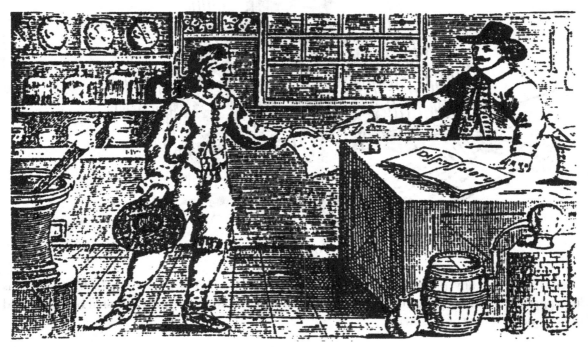

Footnote[230]

For example, Nicholas Culpepper a foremost humane herbalist, of the early eighteen hundreds recommended marijuana goods for improving various medical disorders. To illustrate, he and the Edinburgh New Dispensary explain, when marijuana seeds are in boiled milk and swallowed, it helps with treatments of coughs.[231] Also about this time, the Edinburgh New Dispensary describes, when oil from marijuana seeds is added to milk, "an emulsion is formed, which is useful in treating coughs."[232] Additional information describes, when juice from marijuana seeds is dropped into peoples' or animals' ears, it, "kills worms in them and draws forth earwigs or other living creatures gotten into them."[233] Furthermore, "the emulsion or decoction of the seed: stays lasks and continual fluxes, eases the cholic, allays troublesome humors in the bowels, and stays bleeding at the mouth, nose and other places."[234]

It is also recorded, the decoction of roots from marijuana plants, "allays inflammation of the head, or any other parts, the herb itself, or the distilled water thereof doth the like. The decoction of the roots eases the pains of gout, the hard humors of knots in the joints, the pains and shrinking of the sinews, and pains of the hips. The fresh juice, mixed with a little oil and

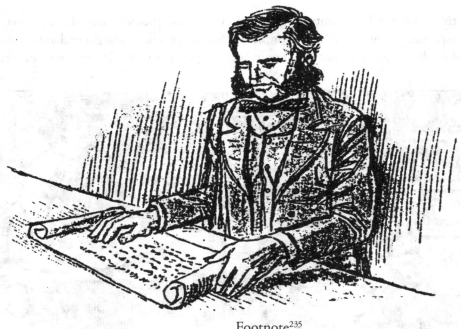

Footnote[235]

butter is good for any place that hath been burnt with fire, being thereto applied."[236] Nicholas Culpepper, in the early eighteen hundreds presented an impressive array of additional beneficial and humane medical uses of marijuana.

Another famous, practical and respected British medical authority, who specifically studied effective medical uses of marijuana was Doctor W.B. O'Shaughnessy. His objective

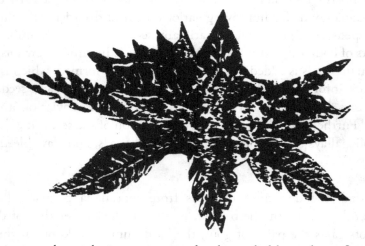

methods, observations and conclusions supported other reliable and confirming reports, about numerous medical benefits resulting from people using or physically ingesting marijuana. It became the, "treatment of choice for vascular or migraine headache (Osler, 1916; O'Shaugnessey, 1839)."[237] During the 1840s, Doctor W.B. O'Shaughnessy administered marijuana to patients, who were suffering from rheumatism. Afterwards, O'Shaughnessy learned many of these patients reported easings of their pains, along with remarkably increased appetites and great mental cheerfulness.[238]

Doctor O'Shaughnessy also used marijuana, in medical improvements and successful treatments for: "cholera, tetanus, and epilepsy, reporting in all cases, his patients experienced relief from the symptoms of these disorders."[239] After testing to ensure marijuana was safe for using with medical patients, Doctor W.B. O'Shaughnessy also prescribed marijuana in a treatment for rabies, with positive results occurring.[240] In addition, Dr. O'Shaughnessy recognized marijuana, "to be an effective analgesic, and to have anticonvulsant and muscle-relaxant properties, which he reported in 1839."[241]

In England (1842) Doctor W.B. O'Shaughnessy and another gentleman, Mr. Peter Squire (a pharmacist) combined information, techniques and resources. Marijuana became processed in such a way, so as to develop a paste that had positive medical properties. This product became known as Squire's Extract.[242] One of the earliest conditions it became successful with was in childbirth. When speaking about this marijuana medical improvement, Doctor John Grigor, a pioneer in obstetrical uses of marijuana found that usually this marijuana medicine, "is capable of bringing the labor to a happy conclusion, considerably within half of the time that would otherwise have been required, thus saving protracted suffering to the patient and time of the practioner."[243] (Humane concern for improved health and welfare were important reasons why marijuana was preferred.) Other medical harms, that Squire's marijuana mixture helped with include: excessive coughing, inability to sleep, migraine headaches, involuntary twitching, pain, loss of appetite, "and treatment of withdrawal symptoms associated with morphine and alcohol addiction."[244]

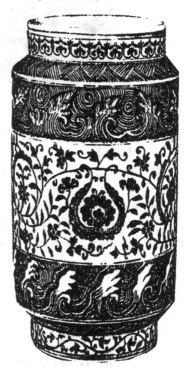

Excessive menstrual bleeding (menorrhagia) became an additional medical difficulty marijuana provided relief for. Doctor Robert Batho, in the eighteen hundreds concluded: marijuana had proven to be, "par excellence the remedy for that condition. . . . It is so certain in its power of controlling menorrhagia."[245] In addition, when speaking about medical uses of marijuana at this time, Doctor John Brown, an English obstetrician humanely concluded, "There is no medicine which has given such good results."[246] It is also recorded, "for at least 3,000 years prior to 1842, widely varying marijuana extracts (buds, leaves, roots, etc.) were the most commonly used, real medicines in the world for the majority of mankind's illnesses."[247] Marijuana provided successful medical treatments for many harmful, "health problems including: asthma, nausea, glaucoma, tumors, epilepsy, infection, stress, migraines, anorexia, depression, rheumatism and arthritis."[248]

Footnote[249]

Trusted doctors found marijuana to be effective treatments for: "alcoholism, dysentery, uterine hemorrhage, migraine, palsy, anthrax, blood poisoning, incontinence, leprosy, snakebite, tonsillitis, parasites, and a legion of other medical problems."[250]

In the United States during the 1800s, millions of marijuana plants and thousands of marijuana plantations freely flourished, without unjust impediments from man-made, restrictive and prohibitive public laws with harmful punishments. Cultivation and constructive uses of marijuana were encouraged by many respected officials, from the Whitehouse to soldiers in battlefields. By 1810, marijuana plants received the accolade of being the, "grand staple of Kentucky."[251] In 1850, 8,327 marijuana plantations were officially recorded in the U.S., largely from Kentucky, Tennessee, Missouri and Mississippi.[252]

Plantations were known to be huge farms with more than 2,000 acres each. Marijuana plants grew successfully and became constructively used in Canada, the United States, Europe

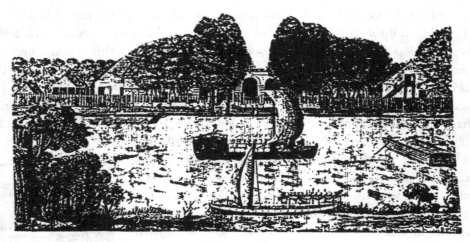

Footnote[253]

and Asia for producing healthy foods, medicines, clothes, shelters, ropes, sails, oils and papers. It became durably known, that marijuana-made sails and clothes resisted damage from winds and sea salt better than any substitute fabric.

Marijuana plants also proved to be effective for making canvas, from the word cannabis, "the rough fabric that covered westward-bound American pioneer wagons."[254] With Clipper Ships and Prairie Schooners, non polluting marijuana plants helped continents of people express

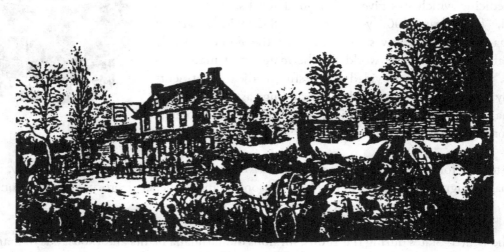

Footnote[255]

their freedoms of liberty, happiness, security and mobility. Environmentally friendly sailboats and covered wagons moved nations of people, natural resources and precious commercial commodities.

Additional useful applications also developed with American made marijuana plants, including being ingredients of fine grade papers, on which were printed official government documents, currencies and contents of Bibles.[256]

Marijuana also grew in America at this time, as a versatile and successful medical resource. The U.S. Dispensatory of 1851 reports preparations of marijuana had been found to: relieve pain, calm spasm, relax nervousness, increase appetite, and improve ability to sleep.[257] Mean and miserable medical harms in the U.S., that marijuana received ongoing improving results for, include: "neuralgia, gout, rheumatism, tetanus, hydrophobia, epidemic cholera, convulsions, chorea, hysteria, mental depression, delirium tremens, insanity, and uterine hemmorhage."[258] Many healthful, humane and trusted medical uses of marijuana became abundantly available in America and numerous other countries around the world, during this time of improving lives, liberty, security, happiness, joy and justice.

The United States Dispensatory, of 1851 also explains that marijuana is *not* a narcotic, like opium. This is because marijuana does not truthfully harm or damage bodily functions, as do real and true narcotics, such as heroin, alcohol, opium or chloral-hydrate. When ingesting or physically consuming true narcotics, truthful harms and damages are done to human bodies, by malfunctioning and inactivating bodily organs and functions, resulting in unhealthy and death-related symptoms such as: diminished appetite, constipation, nausea, and/or failure to sufficiently excrete harmful bodily fluids. With physically consuming marijuana plants, on the other hand, true harms and damages are *not* done to bodies by *not*, "diminishing the appetite, checking the secretions, or constipating the bowels."[259]

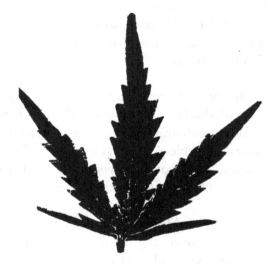

Also, with true narcotics, such as morphine, alcohol, opium or chloral-hydrate, actual, factual and truthful death-related harm is typically done to bodies, by causing additional internal harms, such as headaches and bronchial congestions. Marijuana, however became beneficially and successfully attractive, because it was found *not* to cause headaches, nausea, or bronchial respiratory harms. Marijuana became medically and humanely preferred particularly because, "opium is contraindicated by its nauseating, or constipating effects, or its disposition to produce headache, and to check the bronchial section."[260]

Marijuana also received recognition as being useful for treating people with lockjaw. For example, in New York (1854) a student named Mr. Ludlow observed a container of marijuana, "which the pharmacist advised him was a preparation of East Indian Hemp, considered then to be a . . . remedy for lockjaw."[261]

During this exciting era of improvements, many countries around the world participated in discovering and sharing healthful, medical, industrial, practical and other beneficial information about God's natural green herb marijuana plants.

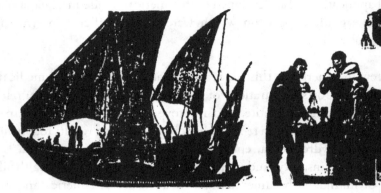

Footnote[262]

Between 1839 and 1900 for example, more than one hundred articles appeared in scientific journals describing nonharmful and medically helpful properties of marijuana.[263] In Germany, marijuana plants were being successfully used for relieving asthma, another difficult medical disorder.[264] Additional developing international countries known to have been successfully and humanely consuming natural marijuana for healthy medical purposes at this time, include: Egypt, Turkey, South Africa, Burma, Siam, the Malays, and South America including Jamaica.[266]

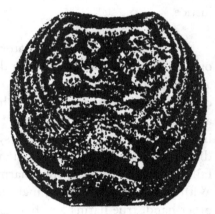

In 1860, Doctor R.R. M'Meens reported on findings of the Ohio Medical Society. Medical disorders listed that marijuana, including its hashish, leaves, buds, seeds, oils, roots and flowers

Footnote[265]

became valuable as medical treatments for include: convulsions, asthma, tetanus, neuralgia, labor pains, chronic bronchitis, gonorrhea, postpartum psychosis and dysmenorrhea, "without interfering with the actions of the internal organs."[267]

The Ohio Medical Society in 1860 also catalogued descriptions of medical harms for which physically consuming marijuana (including its seeds, leaves, buds, oils, roots and hashish resins) provided successful and effective medical results. Among the harmful disorders on this list include: epilepsy, infantile convulsions, whooping cough, muscular spasms, hysteria, mania, nervous rheumatism, palsy, asthma, loss of appetite, tetanus, neuralgia, dysmenorrhea, chronic bronchitis, uterine hemorrhage, and withdrawal from alcohol ingestion.[268] Marijuana was also valued by soldiers in the U.S. Civil War, for many helpful purposes including medical treatments for: diarrhea and dysentery.[269] Multi useful marijuana plant goods were traditionally trusted ingredients in many North American prescriptions, recipes and protective commodities.

The original Declaration of Independence proclaimed by the U.S. federal government in 1776 was also purposely written on marijuana-plant-made paper.[270] In addition, marijuana plants were the

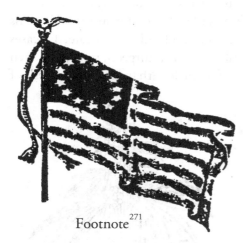

Footnote[271]

natural ingredients with which, "Betsy Ross made the first American flag."[272] When the U.S. federal government adopted the Declaration of Independence, it was felt that a national emblem of union, liberty and independence should be chosen. On June 14, 1777, Congress adopted the following resolution: "Resolved that the flag of the Thirteen United States shall be thirteen stripes alternate white and red, and that the Union be thirteen white stars on a blue field."[273] Betsy Ross, "flag maker residing at 239 Arch Street, Philadelphia made the first flag and suggested that the stars be five-pointed."[274] Philadelphia proudly hosted the emblematic Liberty Bell. At this time, federal government leaders purposely chose marijuana plants as the primary ingredient for making the official paper, on which the original Constitution of the United States was written.[275]

Marijuana oil also developed a popular history for lighting lamps. Until the beginning of the 1800s, marijuana seed oil was the, "most consumed lighting oil in America and the world."[276]

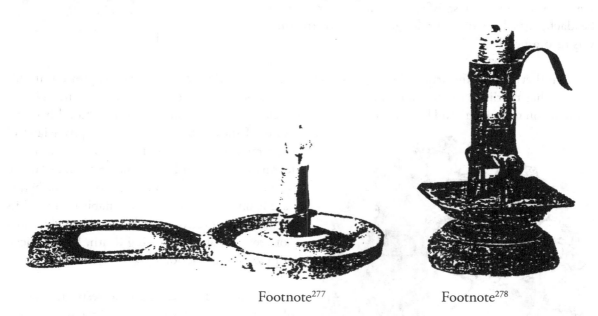

Footnote[277]   Footnote[278]

Oil from marijuana seeds, "lit the lamps of . . . Abraham the prophet and . . . Abraham Lincoln. It was the brightest lamp oil."[279] Multi beneficial marijuana plants developed as an attractive natural resource for making many humane products throughout the world including: China, India, Africa, Arabia, Russia, England, France, Germany, Holland, Ireland, Italy, Japan, Canada and the United States.

By: Joseph W. Jacob B.A., M.P.A.

Doctor J.B. Mattison, a famous U.S. physician during the late eighteen hundreds re-emphasized medical uses of marijuana as a general analgesic and soporific, as well as being an effective medicine for: delerium tremens, migraine headaches, gastric ulcers, asthma, dysmenorrhoea and chronic rheumatism.[280] Dr. J.B. Mattison also found marijuana to be especially effective for curing addictions to true and harmful narcotics such as: morphine, opium, alcohol and chloral-hydrate. In cases involving morphine addiction for example, Dr. Mattison describes, "a naval surgeon, nine years a ten grains daily subcutaneous morphia taker . . . [who] recovered with less than a dozen doses" of marijuana.[281]

In 1889, E. Birch successfully treated a chloral-hydrate addict and another opium addict, with medically using marijuana. In each case Birch observed, "a prompt response, with the return of appetite and sound sleep."[282] In reference to migraine headaches in the United States at this time, Doctor J.B. Mattison further explains that marijuana is not only important in arresting the pain of a migraine headache attack, but it is also useful in preventing such attacks.[283] This humane view received additional medical support from William Osler, whose observations and conclusions explain that marijuana is regarded as the most satisfactory remedy for migraine headache attacks, "and a prolonged course of treatment was recommended."[284]

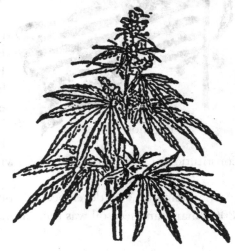

Footnote[285]

Another important truth about physically ingesting marijuana (cannabis) expressed at this time is that marijuana *never* caused death. This is an obvious, significant and actual difference, in comparison to any true and harmful narcotics such as alcohol, heroin, morphine and chloral-hydrate.

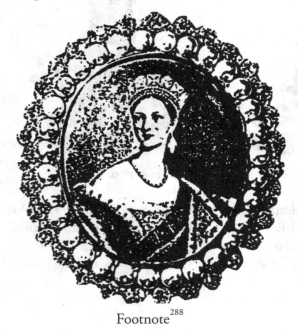

Footnote[288]

Writer Ernest Abel explains how physicians of the time frequently noted while using marijuana (cannabis), "an overdose has never produced death in man or the lower animals. Not one authentic case is on record in which cannabis or any of its preparations destroyed life. . . . Cannabis does not seem capable of causing death, by chemical, or physiological action."[286]

Doctor J.R. Reynolds, a respected court physician to royal Queen Victoria was among prominent British doctors who prescribed and administered marijuana (cannabis), "to his patients."[287] This was perhaps a practical reason why Queen Victoria selected him as her personal doctor. An attractive type of marijuana (cannabis) resin used for medical purposes, before, during and after this time is hashish. "Queen Victoria used cannabis resins for her menstrual cramps and PMS, and her reign (1837-1901) paralleled the enormous growth of the use of Indian cannabis medicine in the English-speaking world."[289] Another reliable source confirms Queen Victoria consumed marijuana goods, including teas, "to relieve her menstrual cramps."[290]

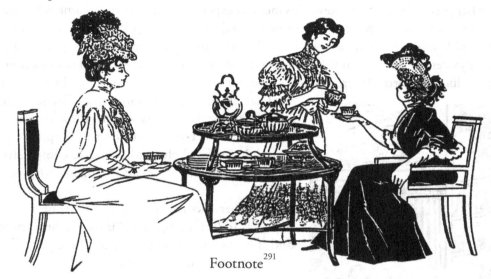

Footnote[291]

Marijuana teas also gained more general medical popularity during this time. Women in particular from Asia and Europe looked forward to and enjoyed precious moments sipping high tea.

Many women received pleasant results from regularly drinking marijuana teas, especially for relieving unpleasant actions in PMS and menstrual cramps. Respected royalty and other knowledgeable people received medical improvements by drinking teas made with leaves, buds, roots and flower tops of green herb marijuana plants. It may well have been that these types of marijuana teas made 'Tea Time' famous in Great Britain and its colonist countries.

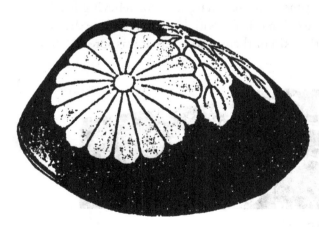

Footnote[294]

Marijuana (including hashish) medically progressed as, "a successful remedy in the treatment of mastitis, dysmenorrhea, menstrual and postpartum pains, and it has been used to increase lactation."[292] In addition, marijuana and hashish extracts were, "the first, second, or third most prescribed medicines in the United States from 1842 until the 1890s."[293]

In 1890, Doctor J.R. Reynolds humanely summarized thirty years of experience he received with marijuana and hash resins. His writings say, "Of the patient with senile insomnia—that is an elderly person who is fidgety at night, goes to bed, gets up again, fusses over his clothes, believes that he has some appointment to keep and must dress himself toward that end—a condition which we at the present time are not always very successful in managing—Reynolds states, "In this class of case, I have found nothing comparable in utility to a moderate dose of Indian hemp."[295] (Indian hemp was known to be cannabis or hashish of the Indica type.)

As another part of Doctor J.R. Reynolds medical experience, marijuana became acknowledged as being, "most valuable in the treatment of various neuralgias including tic douloureux."[296] In addition, Doctor Reynolds found marijuana to be helpful in treating epileptoid states, migraine, depression, asthma and dysmenorrhea.[297] Near the end of the 1800s, respected and educated doctors from around the world, including North America and Europe were using natural marijuana in many beneficial

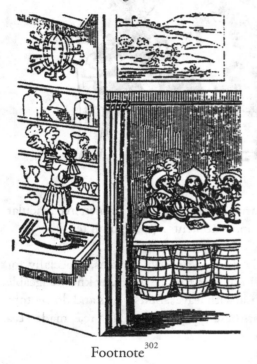

medical treatments for numerous illnesses and other harmful medical disorders. Among those recorded include: sciatica, rabies, tetanus, rheumatism, epilepsy, asthma, neuralgia, melancholy, and obsessive compulsiveness, as well as for anticonvulsant and analgesic purposes.[298]

Another medical report at this time explains that cannabis Indica (marijuana), "is used as an antispasmodic and for its anodyne properties in cases of tetanus, hydrophobia, some forms of mania, etc."[299]

In central Asia at about this time, natural marijuana plants were being eaten, smoked, inhaled, chewed, rubbed onto bodies, sipped with teas and soups, and included in many other helpful mixtures."[300] Doctor Antzyferov wrote a report about Russian uses of marijuana (nasha) around the beginning of the 1900s. He describes that marijuana developed as a successful medication, "for the cure of chronic alcoholics in central Asia."[301] People in Russia at this time also used marijuana for relieving headaches. They mixed marijuana with lamb's fat and ate the mixture

Footnote[302]

with bread, or simply rubbed this mixture onto the skin of their head where it was sore.[303]

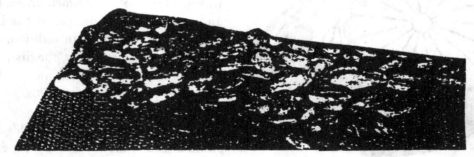

Footnote[304]

In addition, Russian people also made marijuana candies called 'guc-kand' which consisted of marijuana leaves, buds and tops, boiled in water and then put through a sieve, before adding saffron, sugar and several egg whites to it. This mixture was then mashed and formed into several candy-size pieces, before being dried in the sun. Among other things such candies were given to children to keep them from crying. These candies also became a popular treat with women, as it put them in happy moods.[305] Happiness, joy, restful relaxation and improved health were publicly known and trusted attributes of marijuana goods.

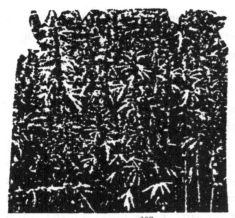

Footnote[307]

Russians also used marijuana for humanely helping animals who were harmed. For example, a cat that had eaten mukhomar (a poisonous mushroom) is placed in a marijuana field to eat marijuana until it, "comes to its senses."[306]

Other areas of Europe and Asia also experienced more help with using natural marijuana for resolving serious medical problems. In Germany, it was learned that by placing sprigs of marijuana on stomachs and ankles of expectant mothers, it would, "prevent convulsions and difficult childbirth."[308]

In Russia, Lithuania and Poland marijuana became medically helpful for alleviating toothaches, by inhaling vapours from seeds that had been tossed on hot rocks.[309] Marijuana resins, buds, leaves and flowers were pressed in and around toothaches for reducing pain, while being an analgesic and disinfectant. Also, in Czechoslovakia, Moravia and Poland marijuana was known as a reliable, humane and trusted treatment for fevers.[310]

In Poland, mixtures of marijuana flowers, wax and olive oil were being successfully, "used to dress wounds."[311] As well, oil from crushed marijuana seeds was found effective in beneficial medical treatments for improving jaundice and rheumatism.[312]

During the late 1800s, numerous substantiated articles were written about many valuable medical uses of marijuana. Trusted reports in related literature describe marijuana's healthful effectiveness for improving an extensive array of medical disorders and diseases. One report from the United States Government, Department of Health, Education and Welfare describes treatments containing marijuana, that became useful for reducing medical harms including: gynecological disorders (as with excessive menstrual cramps and bleeding), migraine headaches, chloral-hydrate addiction, opium addiction, tetanus, insomnia, delerium tremens, muscle spasms, strychnine poisoning, cholera, dysentery, labor pains, psychosis, spasmodic cough, excessive anxiety, depression, gastrointestinal cramps, nervous tremors, psychosomatic illness, bladder irritation and asthma.[313]

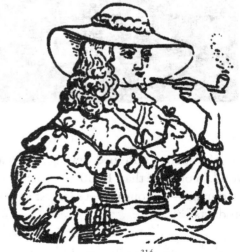

Footnote[314]

Beneficial uses of marijuana for the medical disorder of asthma has been known for many centuries. "The use of cannabis for asthmatics goes back thousands of years in literature. American doctors of the 1800s described in medical papers that, "asthma sufferers would 'bless' Indian Hemp (cannabis) all their lives."[315]

In Argentina, marijuana became beneficial in curative treatments for: cholic, swelling of the liver, gonorrhoea, tetanus, sterility, melancholia, gastralgia, impotency, tuberculosis and asthma.[316]

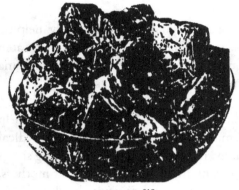

In South Africa at this time, it is recorded that marijuana has, "been used to combat malaria, blackwater fever, blood-poisoning, anthrax and dysentery."[317]

In the United States, marijuana candies progressed into being a favourite and attractive product near the middle of the 1800s. "Starting in the 1860s, the 'Ganjah Wallah Hasheesh Candy Company' made maple sugar hashish candy, which soon became one of the most popular treats in America. It was sold over the counter and advertised in newspapers by Sears-Roebuck, as well as being listed in its own catalogs as a totally harmless fun candy for 40 years."[319]

Footnote[318]

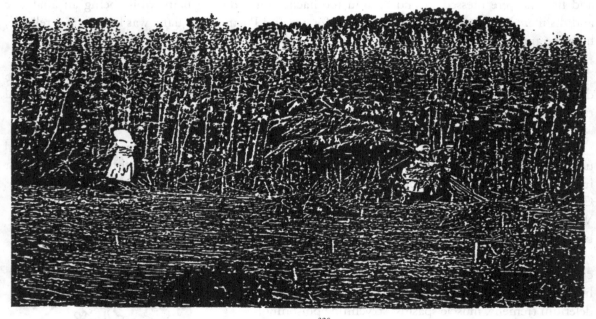

Footnote[320]

Marijuana continued developing as a cherished and valuable natural resource throughout the world. "For more than 1,000 years before the time of Christ until 1883 A.D., cannabis hemp—indeed marijuana—was our planet's largest agricultural crop and most important industry for thousands of products."[321]

At harvest time, many families and friends would gather and help bring in the cannabis crop. It was healthy work that also improved prosperity and social relations. "Whole families came out together to harvest the hemp fields at the height of the flowering season all over the world, for thousands upon thousands of years, never dreaming that it would one day be banned from the face of the earth in favour of fossil fuels, timber and petrochemicals."[322]

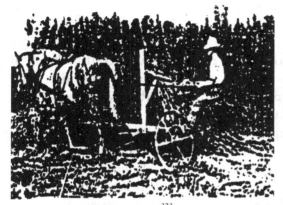

Footnote[323]

By the early 1900s, industrial technology began helping with cultivating and harvesting marijuana plant crops. Both horse drawn mechanical mowers and effective marijuana plant processing machines produced improved output at harvest time.

Writing in 1913, C.J.G. Bourhill also explains that smoking marijuana was not only permitted, but became encouraged among mine workers for improving energy. It is recorded, when smoking cannabis the workers work hard and they, "show very little fatigue."[324] These productive miners were usually allowed to smoke three marijuana cigarettes, during each day at work.

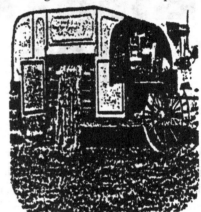

Footnote[325]

In the early 1900s, many immigrants to the United States legally used marijuana as a medical help for relieving respiratory problems. In New York city, for example during the 1920s, it became common for Russian and Polish immigrants to trek over to Nassau Street, buy bulk quantities of marijuana, return to their East-Side tenements, place marijuana on radiators and, "using a towel to form a smoke chamber inhale the fumes for respiratory ailments."[326]

Near the beginning of the 1900s, natural multi-purpose green herb marijuana plants were being cultivated, ingested, transported, bought, trafficked, sold and constructively consumed in legal public democratic freedom throughout Canada and the United States, among many other countries of the world. International patriotic claims of, 'The True North Strong and Free', 'Glorious and Free', and, 'The Home of the Free' appropriately applied to life styles of those who chose to participate in medically using marijuana. It was when liberty meant constructive freedom to add value without harm to people or their property, and without fear of related restriction or harmful punishment. Each year, millions of pounds of natural marijuana plants were being routinely and legally cultivated, harvested, bought, transported, trafficked, sold, imported, exported and publicly consumed by people of all ages.

Naturally grown marijuana plants progressed commercially, domestically and medically, while improving life styles and standards of living for those involved. Many of these participants produced or developed more resistance against diseases, and hence lived longer lives. Using natural marijuana plants had *not* caused even one death, that could be correctly and completely substantiated with authentic, factual, truthful, medical, and/or scientific records, during more than ten thousand continuous years of beneficial public marijuana uses. "In fact, it is invariably reported that no instances of death resulting from the use of cannabis have ever been recorded."[327] (Again, cannabis and hemp were known to be natural, God given green herb marijuana plants.)

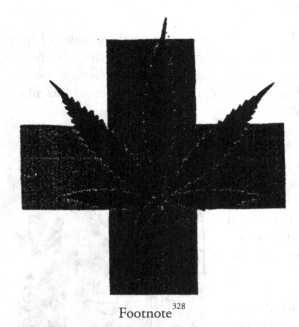

Footnote[328]

During the 1800s, medical uses of marijuana continued increasing as a successful, heathful resource for reducing pains, disorders and discomforts relating to withdrawal from harmful and true narcotics such as: heroin, alcohol, opium, morphine and chloral-hydrate. In addition, marijuana use became encouragingly known to improve and relieve alcohol-related medical disorders including: beri-beri, constipation, cirrhosis, chronic diarrhea and dysentery.

Conversely, ingesting alcohol had been known, shown and truthfully demonstrated to have caused and produced immense amounts of unjustified factual harms, damages, destructions and deaths in Canada, Europe, Russia and the United States. It's not surprising that drinking alcohol produces many demonstrable harms and deaths. After all, alcohol is formed in the liquid that results from death, decay and decomposition of organic products. "No alcohol is found in grapes! No alcohol exists in barley! No alcohol is anywhere found in living plants."[329] The word 'intoxicant' is derived from the Greek word 'toxicon' which means, "the poison into which arrows had been dipped so that their wound might prove fatal."[330]

In early Biblical days, wine often contained *no* alcohol. Homer, a famous Greek writer and poet, who lived about 2,800 years ago wrote of a 'sweet wine' (grape juice) that was first thickened by boiling to which water was then added, before drinking. This wholesome unfermented 'sweet wine' beverage, "contained no alcohol."[331] The boiling process prevents immediate fermentation resulting in no production of alcohol. Similarly, Greeks drank sweet unfermented (or no-alcohol) wine called Gleukos.[332] Also in Egypt reference is made of, "Pharaoh taking the fluid just pressed from the grapes into his cup."[333] Professor Moses Stuart describes the following. "Facts show that the ancients not only preserved their wine unfermented, but regarded it as of a higher flavour and finer quality than fermented wine."[334] It's important to remember, fermented wine truthfully has at least some alcohol in it.

As it seems reasonable to presume that Christ used healthful marijuana plants, it seems equally reasonable to presume that Christ would also have typically used God's healthful unfermented wine, rather than harm producing, fermented alcohol wine. Doctor John J. Owen supports this understanding when he expresses, "As wine was a common beverage in that land of vineyards in its unfermented state, our Lord most likely drank it."[335] A key combination here is 'common beverage' and 'unfermented state'. At this time and place in history, healthful unfermented no-alcohol wine was commonplace with its presence.

Egyptians and Hebrews also drank an unfermented wine called, "tirosh."[336] Doctor Albert Barnes describes additional information supporting the commonality of natural unfermented wine containing no alcohol.

He explains, "The wine of Judea was pure juice of the grape without any mixture of alcohol, and commonly weak and harmless. It was the common drink of the people and did not tend to produce intoxication."[337]

This view is also expressed by Doctor E. Nott who explains, "That unfermented grape juice was called wine is as apparent as it is that it was used as a beverage. It was not only called wine, but it was also accounted to be 'good wine'."[338]

Saint Paul, in his teachings humanely explains, "abstinence from things that are necessarily hurtful to others is a Christian expediency that has the grip of a moral duty."[339]

Further to this subject, Saint Paul carefully advises, "It is good neither to eat flesh, nor to drink wine, nor any other thing whereby thy brother stumbleth."[340] Here, Saint Paul obviously describes alcohol or fermented wine, which throughout history has been known to have caused many brothers to 'stumbleth'.

Louis Pasteur, a famous French scientist discovered that by boiling another organic product, namely milk in an open container (to kill all ferments) and then quickly sealing the

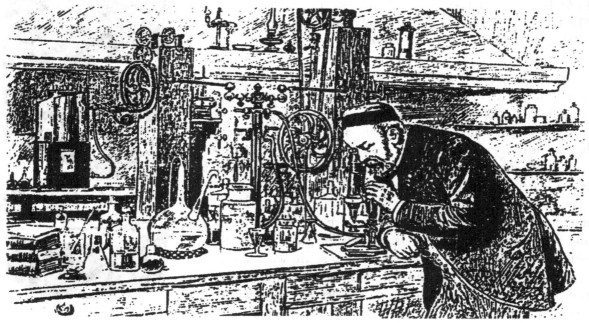

Footnote[341]

container to prevent all other ferments from entering, such boiled and sealed milk would not turn sour. It is nutritiously recorded, "Milk so treated remains perfectly sweet."[342] Similarly, boiling fruit juice in an open container, and then quickly sealing the container eliminates fermentation and alcohol, thereby creating a more nourishing beverage.

A truthful, disgusting and harmful physical feature about alcohol is that it is *not* healthy nutritional food. Doctor Rush (of Philadelphia) published a volume of medical facts regarding the effects of alcohol on human bodies and minds. It was soon, "discovered that alcohol taken into the system was neither digested itself, nor did it help in the digestion of anything else. . . . It was expelled from the system again as alcohol."[343] Simply put, alcohol is not nourishing food, as in *not* adding any medically beneficial nutrients to human bodies and minds.

During the 1900s, North America suffered immense amounts of harms, damages, destructions and deaths due to people (many of them from Christian religions) drinking alcohol. In contrast, other responsible and respected people strived to be industrious, thrifty and self-sufficient, while having good and strong moral characteristics. Many of these people adamantly condemned any and all drinking of alcohol. Consuming alcohol often became associated with lack of personal control, in addition to producing unhappy and harmful results. Mr. A.B. Richmond, a respected and experienced classic American lawyer, when explaining his thoughts about drinking alcohol describes the following, "IT IS THE FOE OF CHRISTIANITY, THE GREAT CAUSE OF POVERTY AND PAUPERISM, THE PROMOTER OF DISEASE AND CRIME, AND SHOULD BE PROHIBITED BY LAW, AND THE LAW ENFORCED BY THE SEVEREST PENALTIES."[344] This obviously was against drinking alcohol, a truthfully proven harm-producer.

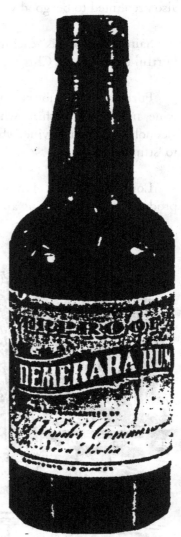

Footnote[345]

Near the beginning of the 1900s in the United States, another intelligent and reliable individual, Colonel Robert G. Ingersoll describes the following effects of people drinking alcohol. It, "cuts down youth in its vigor, manhood in its strength, and age in its weakness. It breaks the father's heart, bereaves the doting mother, extinguishes the natural affection, erases conjugal loves, blots out filial attachments, blights parental hope, and brings down mourning age in sorrow to the grave. It produces weakness not strength, sickness not health, death not life. It makes wives widows, children orphans, fathers fiends, and all of them paupers and beggars. It feeds rheumatism, nurses gout, welcomes epidemics, invites cholera, imports pestilence, and embraces consumption. It covers the land with idleness, misery and crime. It fills your jails, supplies your almshouses, and demands your asylums. It engenders controversies, fosters quarrels and cherishes riots. It crowds your penitentiaries and furnishes victims to your scaffolds. It is the lifeblood of the gambler, the element of the burglar, the prop of the highwayman, and the support of the midnight incendiary. It countenances the liar, respects the thief, and esteems the blasphemer. It violates obligations, reverences fraud, and honors infamy. It defames benevolence, hates love, scorns virtue, and slanders innocence. It incites the father to butcher his helpless offspring, helps the husband to massacre his wife, and the child to grind the parricidal axe. It burns up men, consumes women, detests life, curses God, and despises heaven. It suborns witnesses, nurses perjury, defiles the jury box, and stains the judicial ermine. It degrades the citizen, debases the legislator, dishonors statesmen, and disarms the patriot. It brings shame not honor, terror not safety, despair not hope, misery not happiness, and with the malevolence of a fiend, it calmly surveys its frightful desolation, and unsatisfied with its havoc, it poisons felicity, kills peace, ruins morals, blights confidence, slays reputation, and wipes out national honor, then curses the world and laughs at its ruin. It does all that and more—it murders the soul. It is the son of villainies, the father of crimes, the mother of abominations, the devil's best friend, and God's worst enemy."[346] Alcohol is truthfully concluded to be God's worst enemy.

One of the most abundant types of alcohol being drank in America during this time was rum. Alcohol laden rum was initially imported into America from the West Indies, where purchasing was done with rum. As Mr. Hubert Asbury explains, "At first, the dealers on the African slave coast sold a prime Negro for a few gallons of rum."[347] Demeaning, demonizing and demoralizing alcohol began harming many people, even in North America where laws are supposed to protect people from actual, damaging the truthful harms.

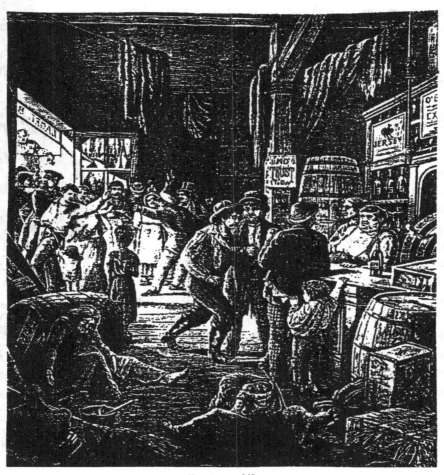

Footnote[348]

By the late 1800s, many people in North America were drinking harmful quantities of rum, in addition to whiskey, gin, beer, vodka and fermented (or alcohol) wine. At this time, Doctor Charles H. Fowler describes bitter, vivid and numerous truthful harms produced by people drinking alcohol. As he explains alcohol, "murders sixty thousand men annually, dooms to an inheritance of rags and shame two millions of children, hangs a millstone around the necks of three millions of women, and casts them into the social sea, sends over two hundred thousand paupers to the poorhouses, and over two hundred thousand criminals to the gallows and the prisons, bequeaths two hundred thousand orphans to public charity, horrifies the year with four hundred and fifty suicides, seven hundred murders, and commits to the demon of lunacy twelve thousand human beings."[349] Alcohol, disgusting conditions, miseries, harms, destructions, poverties and deaths clearly became interrelated throughout many areas of North America.

People drinking alcohol tend to produce many true and factual harmful crimes, while unsuspecting victims suffer several related demonstrable harms. This is as true today as it was during the late 1800s. Damages, miseries and truthfully proven harms from drinking alcohol became known to include: assaults, thefts, arsons, rapes, murders, poverties, laziness, depressions, divorces, destructions, despairs and deaths.

Following are some short, factual and truthful accounts describing demonstrable (or demonstratable) harms, actual damages, obvious destructions and proven violent crimes produced from people drinking alcohol.

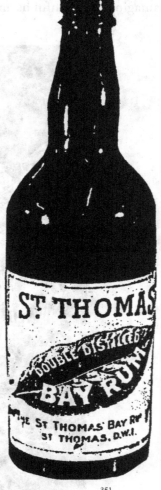

Mr. A.B. Richmond, a respected lawyer from Pennsylvania provides the following courtroom description. "Prisoners at the bar, stand up! said the Judge in cold, authoritative tones. You have been convicted of arson, burglary and aggravated riot. . . . You met together at the hotel of _____, in this county, and after indulging freely in intoxicating liquor, you proceeded to commit criminal acts of violence and incendiarism. You set to fire the house of your employer, and when the proprietor of the hotel very properly refused to give you any more liquor—as you were already intoxicated—and closed his doors against you. You broke into his house, stole his liquor, which you distributed to the mob your unlawful conduct had collected, and when they, like yourselves were drunk and frenzied with intoxicating liquor, you applied the torch of the incendiary to the buildings and workshops where you had been employed. By that act you destroyed a large amount of property, threw out of employment scores of men, who were willing to work, and who depended upon their daily labor for the support of themselves and their families. . . . Your plea, that you were drunk is no excuse in law; it . . . aggravates your crime, for no good law-abiding citizen will get drunk, knowing as every one must know, that men are much more likely to commit crime when they are under the influence of liquor, than when they are sober."[350] A few harmful moments of uncontrolled rage or greed, spurned on with

Footnote[351]

52

drinking alcohol can quickly produce short, medium and long term damages, disorders, disasters and deaths.

Mr. Thomas Trotter L.D.S. describes the following harms occurring to a Canadian family, because of drinking alcohol. These types of alcohol-produced harms afflicted many people in America, including: Native Indians, farmers, merchants, clergy, housewives, children, tradesmen and numerous other typical people. This reputable and factual account begins with Mr. Trotter saying, "I can well remember K., when he was only six months old . . . and the infant took form his mother's hand spoonful after spoonful of the strong unmixed liquor. . . . It was amid the free use of whiskey and its concomitant influences that K. spent his early and advanced boyhood. . . . His mother nursed him until he was over four years old, and one morning while I was delivering a message to her . . . K. ran up to his mother and demanded something in the room from her. . . . Instead of receiving reproof, the little boy received commendation from his mother who said, "Shure, now isn't he a right shmart boy; see how he will have what he wants. . . . The early seeds of intemperance, which had been so well sown in the boy now began to grow apace. His father, when he could obtain it carried with him to his work his little tin of whiskey; of this K. always got a share, and at the end of two or three years it was no uncommon sight after they had received their pay, for Tim and his son to be on a spree together.

At the age of sixteen, K. had become a quarrelsome, swearing besotted drunkard refusing even to assist his father to work, when he could obtain whiskey on which to become drunk; in fact only working to get money for that purpose. The father, who for years had generally kept himself sober enough to work most of the time, now became through age and constant drinking incapable of earning much money, and as a consequence the family was often in a state of want; and the poor wife was often glad to get little jobs of work to earn a shilling, and had often taken the charity of neighbours to save herself from actual want. A few years brought both father and son to the condition of hopeless drunkards avoiding all work save for the purpose of getting it to buy whiskey. . . . K.'s quarrelsome nature, incited by drink had several times got him into prison, and he had become the most degraded and dreaded boy in town, and so heartless were the father and the son, that they made it one of their plans of obtaining liquor to wait around till the wife and mother returned from a day's washing or scrubbing, and forcing her to hand over to them the money she had earned. . . . K. and his father continued in their course of dissipation, until on a certain occasion they returned home about midnight in a drunken state. By some means, K. knew that his mother had saved out of her day's earnings twelve and a half cents, or what was then called 'a York Shilling' and both father and son thirsting for more of the accursed drink demanded the money from her. She refused to give it up, whereupon they both threatened her, but the poor woman again refused to hand over for whiskey the last cent she had to procure her breakfast; and the two then searched the

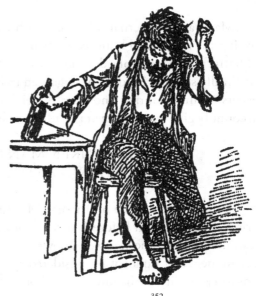

Footnote[352]

house but failing to find the trifle they beat her severely. Search was again made by the two monsters and upon failing the second time, K. took an axe-handle and beat his mother until she had scarcely power of speech left to tell him where she had hidden the York shilling. As soon as he obtained the money, he hurried off and bought a quart of whiskey which he and his father drank, while the woman was lying on the floor outside of her bed, in an insensible state, and they did not awake from their drunken sleep til late in the forenoon. When K. and his father awoke, it was supposed they did not even look into the room where the murdered woman lay, but she was found by a neighbour, breathing her last, while they were found in a tavern and were arrested. . . . The father Tim, who confessed all . . . stated it was the son who inflicted the deadly blows with the axe-handle. . . . When K. was found guilty and asked the usual questions by the judge before passing sentence of death, he remained doggedly silent, and throughout the time that passed before his execution, he showed not the slightest emotion or any sign of repentance. . . . After K.'s execution, Tim, Cain-like wandered about seeking rest but finding none, only when he could get enough whiskey to render himself insensible. He was employed by a Dr. F. to do stable work, and on being missing one night was found in one of the horse stalls near the point of death. The doctor took him in and cared for him, but he soon died."[353] It took awhile, but alcohol with its destructive, cruel, unusual and harmful effects caused death to each and every person in this Canadian family. Many similar damaging results continued occuring throughout North America, as man-made laws promoted drinking alcohol, God's worst enemy.

Truthful harms from people drinking alcohol have grimly damaged and destroyed millions of lives in Canada and the United States. People drinking alcohol since the eighteen hundreds have produced much: unhappiness, vagrancies, demonstrable harms, miseries, pains and deaths, frequently with gruesome circumstances and oftentimes unfairly harming others. By comparison, there are no truthfully substantiated accounts of similar harms produced from people ingesting God's natural green herb marijuana plants at or before this time. Although many fabricated, untrue and fantasy style stories were written to the contrary, for sensationalism and financial gain purposes, it is significant to remember that alcohol's diseases became medically improved with using marijuana, *not* the other way around.

Many actual, factual, hideous, truthful and demonstrable harms produced in North America during the last several hundred years often times include insidious alcohol as a drinkable ingredient of harmful actions. Consider the following typical newspaper account of a reliably documented and truthfully substantiated event, regarded to be similar to at least thousands of other alcohol involved events occuring during and after the eighteen hundreds. This unhappy and tragic alcohol actions account begins with a relevant headline, followed by a specific description of harmful events.

"A DRUNKEN MAN MURDERS HIS WIFE AND LIES DOWN AND SLEEPS BY HER DEAD BODY

A man by the name of Thomas M. was arrested this morning for the murder of his wife. The prisoner was brought before Justice S. for a hearing. He was a very dissipated looking man and the testimony showed he was well known in our community as a common drunkard, and when under the influence of liquor was considered quarrelsome and dangerous. He lived with his wife, in an unsavory locality in the lower part of our city. This morning as officer B. was passing along his beat, he saw a crowd collected in front of a low tenement house, and was informed that one of its inmates had been murdered.

Entering the house, he saw the dead body of the wife of the prisoner lying in a bed, from which it appeared as if the husband had just arisen. An examination of the body proved that the skull had been crushed by a violent blow inflicted with some blunt instrument. The prisoner, partially dressed was seated in a chair by the bedside . . . and stated that when he came home late in the night his wife was in bed crying, that he went to bed and told her to stop her crying, that he could not go to sleep, that she did not stop, and then he got up and struck her with his heavy boot, and then she stopped crying. . . . When he awoke in the morning he found she was dead. . . .

The prisoner was seen late last night very much intoxicated, in a saloon at the corner of S and Fourth streets."[354] Many true, horror-filled, factual and demonstrably harmful accounts exist, all occurring while or after alcohol was being ingested by people.

Alcohol drinking shows no mercy for parents, age or gender as another documented account demonstrates. "One Saturday night the prisoner came home drunk. He was very abusive to his mother, so much so that she left the house and went to a neighbor's. About nine o'clock she returned and found her husband lying dead on the floor, his skull crushed by a cruel blow, apparently given with a stick of firewood. By his side lay the prisoner in a drunken sleep. . . .

The grey hairs of the old man were clotted with blood, and his brains were oozing from his fractured skull. By the side of the son was found a large stick of wood covered with blood and grey hairs. . . . His hands and clothes were stained with his father's blood. But there were the silent, yet truthful evidences of his crime . . . the dead body, the club, and the blood upon his person told the terrible story of his guilt. . . .

The prisoner died in an insane asylum, where he had been taken from the prison, where the solitude of his cell, haunted by the shame of his murdered father had affected his brain—diseased by liquor—and made him a maniac. His poor old mother died heartbroken, before his trial and conviction; and now in a desolate and forsaken graveyard in the country, overgrown with weeds and brambles, father, mother and son sleep side by side—the father killed by the son, and all three indirectly murdered by the law that licenses the sale of intoxicating liquors as a beverage."[356] Cruel alcohol again produced demonstrable harms, miseries, pains and deaths.

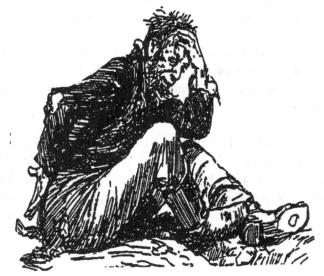

Footnote[355]

By: Joseph W. Jacob B.A., M.P.A.

Since the eighteen hundreds, millions of alcohol produced harms and deaths have occurred in North America and the rest of the world, resulting in considerable true harms to victims, true times for courts, and true costs from taxpayers. About 1880, a prominent U.S. statistician described the annual amount of alcohol-produced-deaths by saying, "In the United States are over seven hundred thousand drunkards, that over one hundred thousand die annually, who go to drunkards' graves, over two hundred and seventy-five die daily, or twelve every hour."[357]

At least one hundred thousand alcohol produced deaths per year multiplied by a hundred years means that drinking alcohol has caused deaths to millions of human beings in North America alone. This obviously contributes to alcohol's bad reputation of being God's worst enemy. By comparison at this time, no similar, truthful and medically or scientifically substantiated, death-producing records resulted from people physically consuming natural marijuana plants.

Women, in particular are oftentimes unfairly treated victims of alcohol produced harms. Assaults, robberies, rapes and murders are special areas of serious concern to women, particularly when alcohol is involved. One author describes how women suffer additional degrading demonstrable harms and damages from behaviours of people drinking alcohol. "Of your number are the thousands and tens of thousands of heartbroken wives in our land, who have lived to see their husbands sacrifice love, home, happiness, reputation and all of life's endearments to the fatal passion for strong drink. Of your number are the multitude of sorrowing mothers, who have mourned over the memory of sons that have gone to drunkards' graves. Of your number are the thousands of poor wives and mothers in our land, who with enfeebled health and weak hands are made to do the labor of the slave to support their families, while the husbands and fathers, drunken and debauched are spending all they can earn in the licenced rum-shop. On your frail bodies fall the brutal blows of the husbands made demonical by rum . . . an evil more destructive to mankind than war, pestilence and famine."[358]

Alcohol is included in many demonstrable harms and deaths. This clear and deceiving liquid is a constant component of numerous public beverages, including: rum, whiskey, beer, brandy, bourbon, gin, fermented wine, home-brew, sake, sherry, port, champagne, vodka, vermouth and various similar liquors.

Alcohol and death are similarly related, first of all because alcohol is formed from death and decay of organic substances. Mr. A.B. Richmond, a practical and realistic American lawyer describes the following relationship between alcohol and death. "A client of mine once called on me to draw his will. He was at that time a man of large property. The will was drawn and left in my keeping. In it he made ample provision for the support of his family and the education of his children.

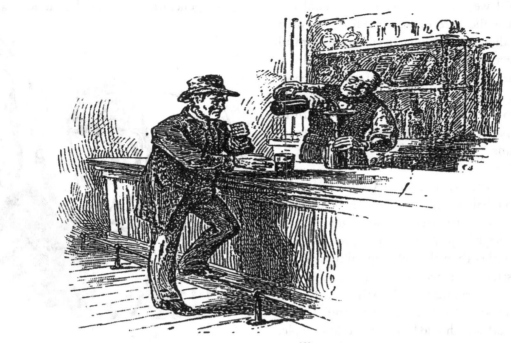

Footnote[359]

Ten years passed away; his property was gone, and he had died a drunkard's death. I stood by his coffin, for he had been my friend, and as the 'dust was returned to dust' I thought of the will he once made and the legacies he now left his family. Yes, I thought of a drunkard's will! It could be written in a few short sentences: "I will and bequeath to my heartbroken wife the memory of broken vows, blighted hopes, penury and woe. I will and bequeath to my little children poverty and shame, and to the rest of my kindred I will and bequeath the recollections of a misspent life and the monument of a drunkard's grave. . . . Go where you will—visit the cities of the dead in every land—and there lie the remains of poets and statesmen, kings and subjects, men of the brightest intellects, as well as of feeble minds—hundreds upon hundreds, thousands upon thousands—yes, millions upon millions filling drunkards' graves, for that demon that hath so long devastated the earth spares neither rich nor poor, plebeian nor patrician, but all alike are its victims."[360] Deceiving alcohol contaminates numerous bodies, minds, souls and graveyards across many American countrysides creating histories of countless demonstrable harms: misery, pain, lonliness, decay, disrespect, disorientation, despair and death. Meantime, man-made laws encourage ingestion of harmful alcohol, while legally prohibiting public ingestion of nonharmful and medically helpful marijuana. Popular constitutional democracies are legally intended to be: *for* the people, by the people, and of the people, where democratic majority-vote rule is official law. This is what legally separates democracies from other dictatorial or tyrannical types of governments. When governments ensure consumption of only nonharmful and nutritionally healthy food for its people, there becomes active and truthful support of government *for* the people. Such humane caring and demonstrably helpful government actions can improve and extend lives for millions of people, while encouraging individuals to be healthy, valuable, nonharmful, peaceful, happy and joyful. Naturally, God prefers healthy rather than harmful food items for people to consume.

"You shall not kill" and "you shall not steal" are two of God's Ten Commandments.[361] These laws of God were given to Moses as moral boundaries for generations of peoples' actions and behaviours while here on earth. However, man made laws allowing its people to consume harmful food products such as alcohol for people to drink and contaminated commercial cigarettes for people to smoke, not only result in more harms to society, but it also steals happiness and health from individual participants, by destroying their internal bodily organs.

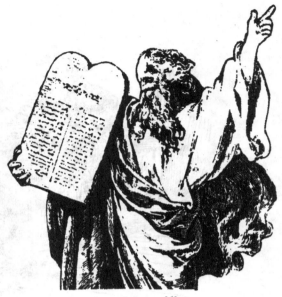

The two extremely important Commandments of God: "You shall not kill" and "You shall not steal" promote peace, order, security, good governance, happiness, health, joy, life, hope, progress and prosperity, rather than alcohol's typical trademarks of demonstrable harms, including: confusions, delusions, destructions, despairs, miseries, pains, poverties, sorrows, tragedies and deaths. Governmental laws should be *for* protecting people, *not* promoting harm to them. Alcohol promotes

Footnote[362]

deaths, while God's green herb marijuana plants and guaranteed constitutional democratic laws advocate: life, liberty, security, protection, happiness and joy for people.

Drinking alcohol not only produces demonstrable harms, of poverties, diseases and deaths, but alcohol also deteriorates a person's health, both physically and mentally. Inside the human body

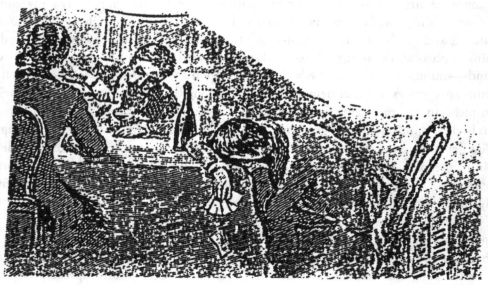

Footnote[363]

alcohol produces an abundant array of demonstrable harms, including medical disorders to the: stomach, brain, liver, pancreas, lungs, heart, kidneys and many other bodily organs. In Stage One, with a healthy non-alcohol-harmed stomach, the mucous coating the stomach is usually slightly reddish in colour, "tinged with yellow."[364] During Stage Two of alcohol-stomach-deterioration to a typical moderate or, "temperate drinker, a man who takes his grog daily but moderately, the effect . . . is to distend the blood-vessels of the inner surface of the stomach, or in other words produce a degree of inflammation which makes the blood-vessels visible."[365] This moderate but daily alcohol drinker, "would be insulted if you were to tell him that there was danger of him becoming a drunkard. He probably is a good citizen, may belong to a church, is a kind husband and father, and has not the remotest idea he is approaching the awful precipice of habitual drunkenness with slow but steady pace. No! He is confident he can command his appetite, despises a drunken sot, and wonders how any man can become so degraded regardless of himself and family, as to become a common drunkard."[366]

When a person drinks alcohol on a daily basis for more than a few years, as with a moderate alcohol drinker in Stage Three of physical deterioration, the stomach, "shows the mucous membrane in a highly inflamed condition. In this state, the inebriate is never satisfied unless the stomach is exited by the presence of alcohol. . . . In this condition, the man is a firm believer . . . that he "must drink no more water." He also believes that it is absolutely necessary for him to take wine or alcohol. . . . At this stage, the drunkard may yet reform and save himself from the terrible tortures of delerium tremens, followed by almost certain death, but it will require a fearful struggle with his appetite, a struggle from which comparatively few come out conquerors. Yet a few, out of the great army of thousands that are marching with steady and certain step to a drunkard's grave do here desert the black flag of death, that floats over that army, and by the exercise of great will power, they do save themselves and become sober men, but the reform is only accomplished by total abstinence."[367] Total abstinence means having *no* alcohol at all in the body at all times. No alcohol at all in the body means no small drink, no special drink, or no any drink or ingestion of any alcohol at any time.

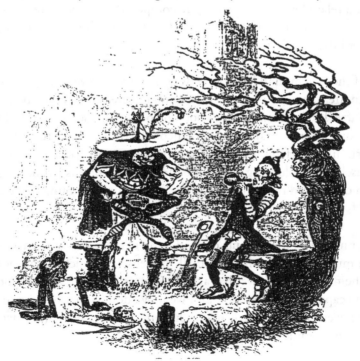

Footnote[368]

In the Fourth Stage of alcohol-stomach-decay and destruction, the inner coat of the person's stomach is typically, "ulcerated as the direct and certain result of alcoholic inflammation. There is yet a faint hope that reformation is possible, but it is not probable. Men have lived and reformed who had arrived at this point on a drunkard's downward career, but not one in a hundred."[369] Less than one in a hundred is very scary odds indeed, but at least it's better than no odds at all as when a person continues drinking alcohol.

During the Fifth and final Death Stage of alcohol-stomach-decay from drinking alcohol, there becomes, "a high degree of inflammation and the color is changed to a livid red."[370] This livid red colour is typically prominent during delerium tremens, and as actual death occurs. The stomach now looks seriously damaged and, "in some places the mucous membrane seems to be in an incipient state of mortification.

The effects of alcohol are not alone seen and felt in the stomach. As soon as it is taken into that organ it excites the heart, through the great sympathetic nerve, quickens its movement in an effort to counteract, through a more rapid supply and change of blood, the local injury being done to the stomach. . . . It also affects the functions of all the organs, hastening and retarding them by turns, thus wasting much of their normal power; it influences the respiratory processes, through the sympathetic and motor nerves. In short, it always in its use sows the germs of an infinity of diseases, and in the end . . . causes death. . . . Not one sentence, not one word can be said or written in its defense, but its effects are always destructive and harmful when used as a beverage."[371] Alcohol deceivingly damages and demonstrably destroys many bodies and minds with much: agonies, cruelness, miseries, pains and sorrows, during the many deterioration processes. In addition to damaging peoples' stomachs, hearts and lungs, alcohol also inflicts much destructive harms to peoples' brains and minds. First of all, human brains and related nerve substances are composed and structured in such a way that they retain alcohol. "Brain and nerve substances specially retain alcohol. . . . Alcohol is in consequence specially destructive to them."[372]

Next, because of the way human bodies are designed, about seven times as much blood typically passes through brain areas, as compared to other average areas of human bodies.[373] When alcohol enters bloodstreams after leaving stomachs, it's not long before alcohol demonstrably harms nerves and tissues of peoples' brains. Even a small amount of alcohol, "though not producing much effect that is visible, still most certainly interferes with the delicacy, correctness and quickness of the action of the nerves upon the muscles, and blunting the mind and the perceptions, while larger doses show their disastrous actions in disordered movements and the rolling and tumbling—the common symptoms of intoxication.

We see then, that muscular movements depend upon nerve power, and that as alcohol injures the nerve it impairs the muscle. Besides this, since all the senses of touch, sight, hearing, smelling and tasting depend on the nerves, it follows that alcohol injures them all, and so not only makes a man less of a man and less capable of enjoyment, and we may add less capable of pain, by blunting every sense and weakening every muscle, but it makes him inaccurate, slow and uncertain, for the nerve system ceases to be able to guide as it otherwise could."[374]

Hang-overs with slow movements, loss of energy, throbbing blood vessels, pounding headaches, dehydration, and irritable attitudes become factual and true typical harmful precipitates of drinking or otherwise ingesting alcohol.

Drinking alcohol also physically deteriorates and produces demonstrable harms to brain cells. Important historic and scientific medical records report how alcohol, "enlarges the cells of the tissues of the brain, that when so enlarged by alcoholic stimulants, they are never again restored to their normal size and condition."[375] Irrepairable damage and weakened body cells may never return to their previous healthy conditions.

Because of this, if a person practises abstinence, by totally stopping drinking all types of alcohol for several consecutive years, and then starts drinking even small amounts of alcohol, once again demonstrable harms soon occur with intensified decaying effects producing more gruesome pains and deaths.

Even, "after long years have elapsed and the reformed inebriate believes he has conquered his enemy, a single drink will revive the craving in all its former fury."[376] Brain cells not only retain alcohol, but they also degenerate into disfigured shapes of irreparable matter when alcohol is included. Demonstrably harmful, disgusting, horrific and true are the ill, evil and vile results of alcohol drinking.

In addition to truthfully harming brains and stomachs, alcohol also demonstrably harms peoples' livers. "The most common effect of alcohol is to kill numbers of the liver cells and harden them, so the whole organ swells and becomes solid in texture and pale in colour."[377]

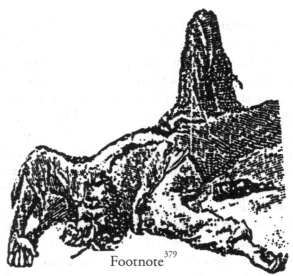

Footnote[379]

After the liver becomes demonstrably harmed, other interrelated bodily organs soon begin malfunctioning. "The importance of the liver is so very great, that when it is disordered the whole body is more or less deranged."[378] Impurities gather as liver and kidney organs fail to filter and clean as they should, or once did. Related harmful irritations then affect important breathing and digestion areas of peoples' bodies. "Alcohol as in the stomach, so in the liver irritates and inflames, and . . . at last destroys."[380] Cirrhosis is but one resulting harmful disease.

The following explanation describes substantiated effects of alcohol on peoples' lungs, kidneys and respiratory processes. "The lungs are irritated, the delicate membrane of the air cells is thickened, and the work of oxygenating the blood thus made more difficult. The engorgement of the blood vessels, and the weakening of the controlling nerves predisposes to bronchitis and inflammatory disorders of the chest. . . . The kidneys, in the same way are not only damaged, but also made peculiarly liable to attacks of various forms of disease."[381]

Drinking alcohol not only destroys human organs, but it also spawns numerous diseases. Early in the 1900s, a prominent American medical professor, Doctor Thomas Sewell was asked what diseases are produced from people drinking alcohol. He knowledgeably responded, "Dyspepsia, jaundice, emaciation, corpulence, rheumatism, gout, palpitation, epilepsy, lethargy, palsy, apoplexy, melancholy, madness, delerium tremens, and premature old age compose but a small part of the endless catalogue of diseases produced by alcohol-drinking."[382]

Alcohol also reduces the ability of human bodies to withstand cold temperatures. Doctor Kane, in an Arctic expedition found that sailors who drank no alcohol, "could best withstand the terrible cold of that region."[383] He also personally learned, that ingesting alcohol caused his body to lose its ability to resist cold temperatures. When discussing effects of alcohol reducing human physical and mental endurances, Doctor N.S. Davis of Chicago concludes, "The use of alcoholic drinks diminishes man's capacity to endure both mental and physical labor, increases a person's predisposition to disease, and shortens the average duration of life."[384] Doctor W.B. Carpenter similarly medically observed and decisively concluded, "Alcohol cannot supply anything which is essential to the . . . nutrition of the tissues."[385] In other words, alcohol is not nutritional food. Instead, drinking alcohol produces true and substantiated demonstrable harms including: decay, disease, discomfort, inactivation, impairment, pain, strain, sterility, misery, unreliability, weakness, disrespect, lonliness, coma and death.

One harmful disease resulting from drinking alcohol is delerium tremens. Doctor Thomas Trotter describes it, "as one of the most terrible calamities which can befall a human being. The whole system is disordered and in a complete state of unrest, the stomach abhors food and the victim is unable to obtain a minute's sleep. Add to this physical condition the fact that the mind is tortured with the most vivid conceptions of everything that may be truly called horrible—the distorted vision of pictures, the most fearful forms and figures in the simplest objects."[386] Doctor Trotter describes a case of delerium tremens involving a prosperous, educated and promising man, who was introduced to drinking alcohol by his family and friends, and thereafter become accustomed to drinking at least some alcohol every day. This alcohol-drinking person, known as R.M. began complaining about nasty mental strains including being, "constantly haunted by various unpleasant scenes and sights. . . . At such times, he seemed to be speechless with terror. After one of those silent periods, he thought a door opened into another room, and there stood grinning at him, a fearful-looking being with a shovel in his hand. The figure said to him, "I'll give it to you now" and began to throw into the room, heaps of vermin with the shovel. The poor fellow immediately jumped out of his bed, weak and trembling and shouted, "They are on me, they are on me," and ran about the room trying to rub the vermin off his body. . . . Again, another door opened, on what appeared to him as an immensely large hall, so dimly lighted that he could barely discover the outlines of some inhuman figures, through their countenances, which were lighted by a horrible glare of bluish light. One of those figures approached the door and grinning at my charge said, turning to the figure behind him, "We will test him on the snake question now." The sufferer then thought that the 'horrid gang' as he called them disappeared, to return in a few minutes bearing on their shoulders a monster snake, thirty feet in length, the eyes of which were flashing bluish beams of light and its tongue shooting out. . . . Then he thought they placed the snake over the footboard of his bed, the head coming up to near his chin and tongues of fire surrounding his head.

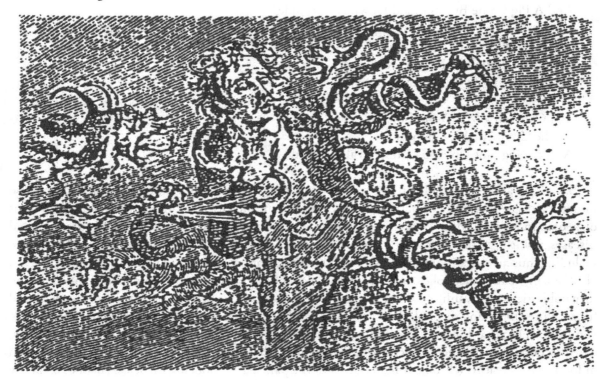

Footnote[387]

The man's whole body shook and his face was a literal picture of despair. . . . The monster snake was again placed in its former position and immediately there issued from its huge mouth thousands of little snakes, which crept under the bedclothes, into the victim's ears, nose and mouth, and finally a large snake curled itself around his neck and tried to choke him."[388] In many stressful cases, horrors and strains along with fears and exhaustions produced from people drinking alcohol result in more serious medical harms including: insomnia, heart attack, stroke, loss of appetite, constipation, unconsciousness, coma and death. Such are the destinies of those who drink alcohol, God's worst enemy. Again in stark contrast, no similar truthful and substantiated harmful accounts were reliably recorded resulting from people ingesting marijuana during this same continuous time span of at least four hundred years. No harmful effects from God's natural green herb marijuana is rather impressive, especially when compared to multi-harmful alcohol-drinking.

Drinking alcohol also causes losses of control, dignity and respect, amid a vast chaotic array of other demonstrable harms. Even pigs don't like alcohol, as the following poem suggests.

On an Evening in October
When He Was Far From Feeling Sober
And Stumbling Slowly Home From Side to Side

By: Joseph W. Jacob B.A., M.P.A.

His Feet Began to Stutter
So He Laid Down In A Gutter
And A Pig Came By And Laid Down At His Side

As He Laid There In the Gutter
Thinking Thoughts He Dare Not Utter
A Lady Passing By Was Heard To Say

You Can Tell a Man Who Boozes
By the Company He Chooses
And the Pig Got Up And Calmly Walked Away

Drinking alcohol not only produces stumbling, staggering, insensibilities and deaths, but it also mutates a disgusting array of harmful medical disorders and diseases, miserably afflicting millions of people in society. More than 150 different harmful and medically substantiated disorders and diseases resulting from ingesting alcohol include: nerve and muscle damage causing weakness, including muscular dystrophy, paralysis and burning sensations in feet and hands, alcoholic hepatitis, alcoholic myopathy, alcoholic cardiomyopathy, alcoholic hypoglycemia, alcoholic hyperlipemia, and megaloblastic anemia, infiltration of the liver with fat (Fatty Liver), cirrhosis, cancer of the liver, and liver failure. Drinking alcohol also truthfully produces gastrointestinal harms including: nausea, vomiting, refluxing, hiccuping, esophagitis, esophageal carcinoma, and cancer of the esophagus, gastritis, cutaneous and peptic ulcers, diarrhea, chronic diarrhea, dysentery, and impaired absorption of food or pancreatitis (chronic inflammation of the pancreas) producing diabetes. Alcohol certainly is *not* nutritious food.

Additional alcohol-produced medical harms affecting peoples' skin, neurology, psychiatry, and respiratory processes include: scurvy, pellagra, alcoholic hallucinosis, Parkinson's Disease, speech impairments, bronchitis, tuberculosis, convulsive disorders, telangiectasia, rhinophyma, peripheral neuropathy, rosacea, and constipation. More typical medical harms produced from drinking alcohol include: malnutrition from reduced intake of food, toxic effects of alcohol on intestines, anorexia, and dehydration resulting in weight-loss with some people and impaired metabolism. Peoples' endocrine systems also become physically harmed from drinking alcohol, with overproduction of cortisol, producing obesity. Alcohol consumption can increase acne, anxiety, palpitations, sweating, headaches, migraine headaches, and tremors, along with a fall in blood-sugar, sometimes producing coma and even death. Other substantiated medical harms developed from drinking alcohol include: high blood pressure (leading to cardiovascular disease) kidney damage, abnormal heart rhythms, pneumonia, blood clots, strokes, fevers, and heart attacks. Additional health harms happening from having alcohol are: subdural hematomas and extradural hematomas, which are effusions of blood between the skull and the brain, usually resulting from head injuries. Drinking alcohol also produces other demonstrable harms to peoples' brains, including mental confusions and nonprogressive intellectual impairments, as with: Korsakoff's Syndrome, retrograde amnesia, cerebral degeneration and dementia.

More medical harms from drinking alcohol include: fractured ribs, hallucinations, fits, delerium tremens, and chronic heart muscle damage (leading to heart failure). Other alcohol induced medical harms include: impaired vision (as with double-vision and focus problems), impaired balance (as in staggering, stumbling and rolling), impaired touch-feelings, insensibilities to pains and related harms, impaired taste abilities, lethargy and fatigue, tooth decay, and impaired smell capabilities. In addition, alcohol drinking causes slow healing from injuries. Reproductive systems are also damaged from drinking alcohol. For women, menstruation irregularities occur, as well as shrinkage of breasts, lactation reduction, and shrinkage of external genitalia. With men, alcohol drinking reduces potency, while shrinking sizes of testes and penis, and losing sexual hair.

Alcohol-drinking also results in reduced or absent sperm formation followed with infertility and sterility. Drinking alcohol is known to demonstrably harm fetuses as with Fetal Alcohol Syndrome. Alcohol in children causes: depressed respiration, low blood-sugar levels, dehydration, hypothermia, coma, and sometimes death. Drinking alcohol is also truthfully known to reduce effectiveness of otherwise helpful medicines, and increase chances of producing harmful side-effects from prescribed drugs. In addition, drinking alcohol impairs work performance and decision making, while increasing safety risks and severity of accidents. It is also reported, "eighty percent of individuals with alcoholic cardiomyopathy, who continue to drink are dead within three years of diagnosis."[389]

Substantiated medical records further show that drinking alcohol directly inhibits glucose synthesis from amino acids, thereby harming nutritional processing functions of the body. Alcohol-drinking is likewise reported to blunt control of the thyroid function by the hypothalamus. Failure to frequently provide essential nonharmful nutrients to human bodies produces deterioration of peoples' organs and immune systems, which can expose them to even more risks of medical harms and diseases including: immune deficiency, dissipation and leprosy.

Trying to reduce demonstrable harms from people drinking alcohol developed into an international moral issue, with courageous efforts from people in the United States, Canada and England. About 1880, a prominant and persistent U.S. female leader Frances E. Willard reported many horrors from people drinking alcohol, and its cruel, harmful, immoral and gruesome effects are very similar today. Frances E. Willard concludes, "Seventy-five per cent of all murders in the country are committed through the influence of rum, fifty per cent of all insanity in the country is the result of drinking, eighty-six per cent of all criminals in the land become such while staggering under a load of liquor, ninety-six per cent of all drunken youths leave a fond but agonized mother's arms to go to the black perdition of strong drink. Every year 100,000 of our best and brightest men reel into eternity and a drunkard's grave.

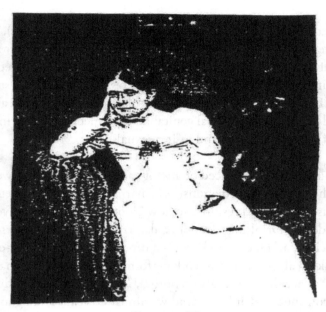

Footnote[390]

Every year, statistics tell us of 500,000 steady drinkers and a million moderate drinkers, and last of all there are millions of handsome intelligent lads going tramp, tramp, tramp to a drunkard's destiny."[391]

Alcohol has truthfully been North America's largest, most harmful and most expensive public menace for at least the last 200 years. Whereas, natural green herb marijuana promotes life as with: medicines, foods, shelters, clothes and respect, conversely alcohol produces many true and demonstrable harms including: diseases, deaths and disrespect.

John Adams, second President of the United States wrote to a friend explaining his disgust and utter disregard for people drinking alcohol. President Adams describes how he became, "fired with a zeal amounting to enthusiasm against ardent spirits, the multiplication of taverns . . . dramshops and tippling houses, and grieved to the heart to see the number of idlers, thieves, sots and consumptive patients made for the physician."[392]

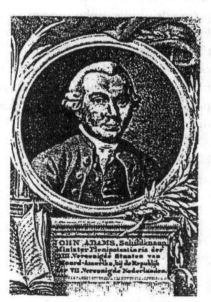

People continually drinking alcohol kept causing costly crimes, harms and damages. Finally, many concerned and reasonable individuals, within the democracy of the United States bravely stepped forward and organized methods for stopping people from drinking or physically ingesting alcohol. The first national organization to discourage people from drinking alcohol in America appeared in Massachusetts, in 1826. It was called the American Society for the Promotion of Temperance.[393] A primary purpose here was to reduce the amount of alcohol being physically ingested by people in America.

Footnote[394]

Another serious effort for democratically reducing amounts of alcohol being drank by people in the United States occurred in 1829, with an official proclamation of Maine's local option law, which allowed each of its counties, "to vote itself 'wet' or 'dry'."[395] Dry meant it was unlawful for people to drink alcohol, while wet meant it was legal for people to ingest alcohol. In 1846, Maine passed its state-wide Prohibition Act, and by 1865 following the U.S. Civil War, thirteen different U.S. States had similar alcohol prohibition protection laws. In 1874, with leadership from Frances E. Willard and Carey Nation, the Woman's Christian Temperance Union (WCTU) established in the United States having a persistant objective of reducing alcohol-drinking in America. By 1900 in the U.S., the 'dry' fight against people drinking alcohol continued receiving public support, especially from many small towns, churches and rural politicians who constantly encouraged increased moral thinking.

Leadership for this 'dry' fight, or public reaction against people drinking alcohol, also came from a fairly new but effective and well-intentioned organization known as the Anti-Saloon League.

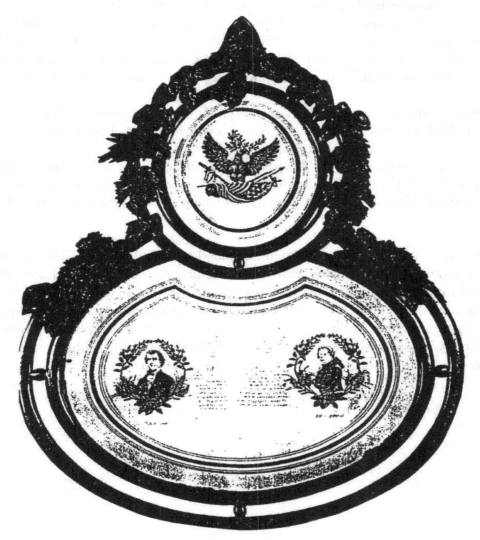

Footnote[396]

By the beginning of the 1900s, "approximately 23% of all Americans lived in 'dry' areas."[397] Nearly a quarter of the country legally received substantial security and protection, rather than being innocent victims of numerous severe harms from destructive and violent people drinking alcohol.

Compelling economic and health reasons were also officially presented in the United States to help stop alcohol-drinking. Industrial areas of the country began observing that alcohol drinking workers were known for doing more demonstrable harms at their workplaces than was expected. Again, from a comparative point of view it's interesting to note that no similar, truthfully-substantiated, demonstrable-harm-concerns were publicly expressed and recorded about people who regularly ingested marijuana goods. Reputable and official organizations, such as the Knights of Labor (a prominent American trade union) presented no similar records or reports against people who routinely ingested marijuana goods during this time of liberty, or freedom to add value without harm.

Economic reasons for legally prohibiting people from drinking alcohol were directed towards two large industrial groups: employers and employees. Four important public alcohol drinking security concerns emerged: safety, stability, punctuality and discipline. During the 1880s and 1890s, the Knights of Labor developed a 'stay-dry' attitude with workers and related influential organizations, while also encouraging the public to avoid drinking alcohol because of its many harms.

In efforts for reducing demonstrable-harms and problems resulting from people drinking alcohol, the Knights of Labor waged a campaign for its members against alcohol-drinking.[398]

Other societies, organizations and churches also began supporting drives against drinking and trafficking of alcohol. Catholic, Baptist and Methodist churches, for example continued advising people to avoid evils of drinking alcohol. The Catholic Church even created its own 'Total Abstinance Society'.

To these reasonable and concerned citizens, alcohol-drinking caused many demonstrable-harms including: assaults, thefts, rapes, destructions, fires, poverties, miseries, pains and deaths. Meanwhile in America during this continuous four hundred year time span, not even one society or reputable organization officially criticized or condemned people for physically consuming, smoking, eating or otherwise ingesting marijuana. No truthfully-substantiated and reliable organizations were recorded as ever having been harmed from smoking, eating or otherwise ingesting marijuana/cannabis/hemp during this time range of more than four hundred consecutive years.

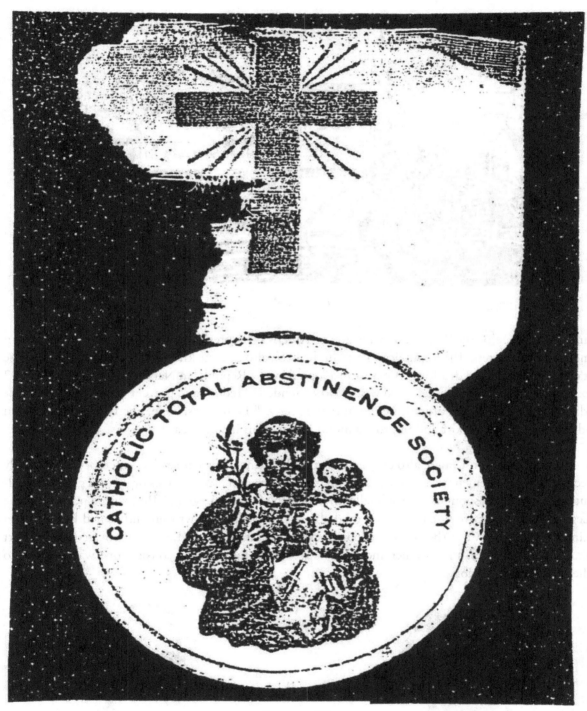

Footnote[399]

On December 17th and 18th 1895, a convention was held at Calvary Baptist Church in Washington D.C., where forty-seven national, state and local organizations agreed to amalgamate their efforts against drinking and trafficking of alcohol. They collectively merged

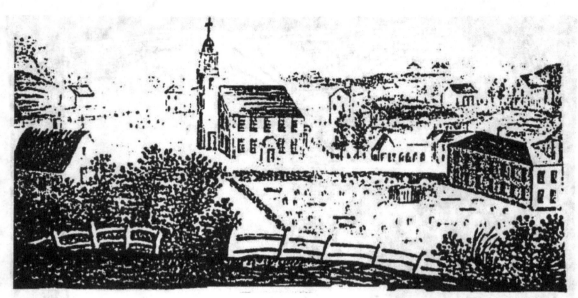

Footnote[400]

under the name of the Anti-Saloon League of America. Its president, Mr. Price was a Republican member of Congress. The Republican Party in the U.S., also became known as the 'dry' party, because it condemned alcohol drinking. A platform adopted by the Republican National Convention of 1892 expressed support for all honest and wise efforts intended to reduce and prevent evils of intemperance (drinking alcohol) while promoting morality in society.[401] Happiness, hope, liberty and logic created additional public support and improved moral momentum in America.

The Anti-Saloon League also created a 'Total Abstinence Department'. It's members continually received encouragement to avoid drinking any and all types of alcohol. This organized group of well-intentioned people soon became officially known as the Lincoln Legion. "The avowed purpose of the Legion was to procure signatures to a total abstinence pledge . . . written and signed by Abraham Lincoln, in 1846. When the South failed to display much interest, the League discovered that Robert E. Lee had also been an abstainer and a firm advocate of temperance, so the name was changed to the Lincoln-Lee Legion.

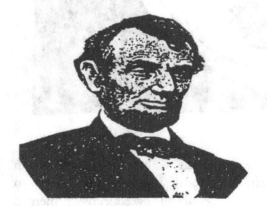

Footnote[402]

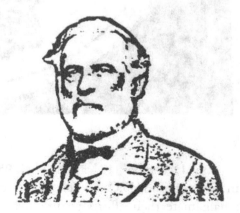

Footnote[403]

By 1916, the Legion had obtained some 3,500,000 pledge signers."[404] Many responsible, respected and reliable individuals unequivocally understood that people continually drinking alcohol produce numerous cruel, true and serious demonstrable harms, including destructions, diseases, poverties and deaths throughout the world. Drinking alcohol, internationally known for producing aggressions, harms and murders was legally and abundantly available in most countries that fought and killed each other during World War One (1914—1918). Alcohol, aggressions, greed and willingnesses to kill other people all wound into a wretched web of wicked reasons why wasteful World War I was woefully waged.

In the United States however, active public sentiment increased support for legal prohibition of alcohol, because of its involvements with many substantiated, unhappy situations and demonstrable harms including: miseries, agonies, despairs, diseases and deaths. It is recorded, "by 1919, before the passage of the 18th Amendment, an additional 19 states passed restrictive legislation, and more than 50% of the U.S. population lived in dry areas."[405] By January 1920, legislated prohibition of alcohol, "was already in effect in 33 states covering 95% of the land area and 63% of the total population of the United States. . . . In 1917, the Hobson Resolution for submission of the Prohibition Amendment to the States received the necessary two-thirds vote in Congress, the Amendment was ratified on January 16, 1919 and went into effect on January 16, 1920. The text of the Amendment was as follows:

Section 1. After one year from the ratification of this article, the manufacture, sale, or transportation of intoxicating liquors within, the importation thereof into, or the exportation thereof from the United States and all territory subject to the jurisdiction thereof, for beverage purposes is hereby prohibited.

Section 2. The Congress and the several States shall have concurrent power to enforce this article by appropriate legislation.

Section 3. This article shall be inoperative, unless it shall have been ratified as an amendment to the Constitution, by the Legislatures of the several States as provided in the Constitution, within seven years from the date of the submission hereof to the States by the Congress."[406]

For many thousands of consecutive years, natural green herb marijuana plants (cannabis/hemp) provided a vast array of healthy foods and medicines, along with paper, secure shelters, and clothing for millions of constructive people attempting to improve their life styles and surroundings.

By: Joseph W. Jacob B.A., M.P.A.

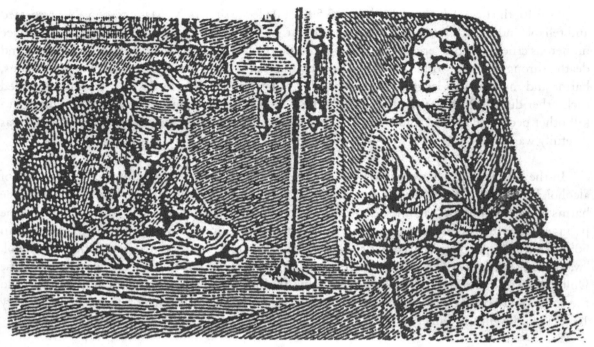

Footnote[407]

Similarly, several serious and sacred religious ceremonies relied on using nourishing natural green herb marijuana. In truthful contrast, during this same extensive continuous time span, alcohol became morally described as God's worst enemy, because of alcohol's consistent involvement in many true and violent demonstrable harms. By 1920, millions of Americans had democratically voted to prohibit manufacturing and selling alcohol for drinking purposes. Also by 1920, these same Americans did not regard marijuana as being harmful. The American public democratically voted and denounced alcohol drinking, because of its demonstrably harmful results. However, regarding the truth, the whole truth and nothing but the truth, it is a true fact that no specific, public, democratic, national referendum, or plebiscite has ever been officially conducted in Canada or the United States, that legally approved public prohibition of nonharmful marijuana uses.

During the late 1800s and early 1900s, some influential medical personnel began changing their prescriptions from naturally grown marijuana medicines to more inorganic multi-chemical pharmaceuticals, many of which have been known and shown to have demonstrably harmful side-effects and inferior beneficial medical effectiveness.

As alcohol-drinking expanded into a huge substantiated public menace throughout the world, marijuana plants provided an impressive array of beneficial public medical uses, among several other constructive improvements. In fact, marijuana became effectively useful during this time for relieving and resolving many public medical disorders, including demonstrable medical harms produced from people drinking alcohol. Alcohol drinking, a true and substantiated public menace continued causing diseases, discomforts, disorders and deaths, while marijuana helped with improving: lives, security, comfort, happiness, protection, nutrition, liberty and joy for multi millions of prudent people.

CHAPTER FOUR

SECRETS OF DISCRIMINATION

MANY MEDICAL BENEFITS WITH MARIJUANA PLANTS WERE SUDDENLY AND SECRETIVELY LEGISLATED FROM SOCIETY *WITHOUT* PUBLIC APPROVAL AND *WITHOUT* MEDICAL JUSTIFICATION (1923-1937)

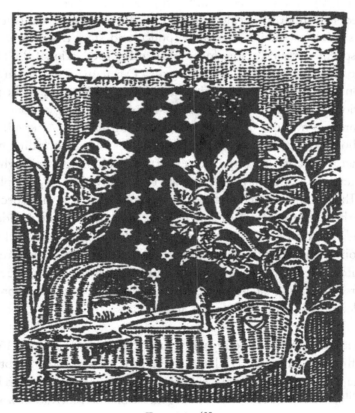

Footnote[408]
Legal prohibition of alcohol in the United States was fit for failure, before the end of the first year of federal enforcement efforts. At least two important incomplete requirements developed, that would

By: Joseph W. Jacob B.A., M.P.A.

soon lead to the demise, disintegration and downfall of this national alcohol prohibition legislation. The first significant deficiency of these alcohol prohibition laws was observed in Section 1 of the National Prohibition Act itself. Obvious, because of its absence was no clause prohibiting people from drinking alcohol. Even though, a primary initial intention of this prohibition act was to stop people from drinking alcohol, there was no actual clause to this effect in the proclaimed act. Section 1 of the National Prohibition Act stated that the manufacture, sale, transportation, importation or exportation of intoxicating liquors for beverage purposes was prohibited. Nothing specified that the actual drinking of alcohol was legally prohibited. In fact, not only was nothing stated about it being unlawful for people to drink alcohol, but also nothing was proclaimed in the U.S. National Prohibition Act of 1920 that prohibited people from giving alcohol for drinking purposes to other people such as delinquents and children, for example. It was only unlawful to manufacture, sell, transport, import or export intoxicating liquors. Nothing prohibiting a person from drinking alcohol or giving alcohol for ingesting purposes to another person was ever stated in this U.S. National Prohibition Act. Incomplete legislation soon produced more truthful demonstrable harms.

Insufficient enforcement specifications also prevented this prohibition legislation from becoming effective. Unorganized procedures and resources were made available for enforcing this National Prohibition Act. Section 2 of the act declared, "The Congress and the several States shall have concurrent power to enforce this article by appropriate legislation."[409] However, appropriate enforcement legislation was never correctly and completely described or implemented, that would effectively prevent people from drinking alcohol. First of all, typical state and federal law enforcement agencies and officers, such as sheriffs, marshals, police and state troopers were not individually mandated, or given specific responsibilities for implementing the National Prohibition Act. Instead, "the Commissioner of Internal Revenue of the Treasury Department was given the power to detect and suppress violations."[410] Having the Commissioner of Internal Revenue as the person mandated to enforce the U.S. National Prohibition Act was unusual. First of all, how was one person and his small bureau expected to prevent millions of people from drinking alcohol? After all, it was known to be the drinking of alcohol that contributed to producing violent harms, including murders and deaths, not the sale, manufacture, transport, import or export of alcohol. Secondly, what expertise did the Commissioner of Internal Revenue have that applied to actually changing peoples' eating, drinking and health habits? The Commissioner of Internal Revenue was typically specialized in receiving taxation money for the U.S. federal government, not conducting country-wide policing activities involving alcohol and transportation. Changing peoples' drinking and health habits more logically fell within jurisdictions such as health, education or consumer affairs. Dismal results of initially co-ordinating appropriate and effective legislation, enforcement resources, and practical procedures for prohibiting people from drinking alcohol were the main reasons why public prohibition of alcohol flatly faltered, fumbled and failed in the United States.

From its first fickle feebleness floundering with faulty leadership on January 16, 1920 the National Prohibition Act was flirting with failure. In January 1920 the New York Sun quoted Daniel C. Roper (Commissioner of the U.S. Federal Internal Revenue) as saying, "The prohibition Law will be violated —extremely at first."[411] Insufficient enforcement, organization and motivation would soon contribute to corruption, disrespect and dissolvement of this official national alcohol prohibition law. "The Prohibition Unit as finally organized comprised 1,520 enforcement agents, or approximately one to every seventy thousand of the population. Nearly all were paid less than two thousand dollars a year, and most received the minimum of $1,680. All authorities agreed that it was impossible for a man, with a family to live decently on these salaries in any large city in the country."[412]

Another report concludes, "Within a year the problems of enforcement were obvious: the diversion of industrial alcohol, congestion in the courts, police lassitude, unwillingness of states to share enforcement with the federal government, governmental corruption, insufficient funds and political hypocrisy.

The law led to seizures of property, violence and even killings by those whose task was to supervise it."[413] This additional alcohol menace added more truthful harms in America, above and beyond the millions of deaths that had already resulted from people drinking alcohol.

The Canadian federal government collected additional taxation revenues with alcohol sales resulting from prohibition in the United States. Although, additional alcohol related deaths became evident from alcohol prohibition in the United States, the Canadian federal government did not enact any national alcohol prohibition legislation in Canada. Instead, by doing nothing the government of Canada continued collecting multi millions of additional tax revenue dollars annually, especially from alcohol destined to the U.S. While cunningly collecting this big time easy money, political attention was changed to another area.

During the early 1920s, the Canadian federal government and legal system, without substantiated justification, suddenly began condemning God's most preferred plant, green herb cannabis (or soon-to-be, marijuana) for allegedly causing society's damages and crimes. The same harmful features, previously well known about alcohol, God's worst enemy, suddenly and without truthful substantiation were being applied against helpful marijuana plants and people who nonharmfully used them.

By not expressing official concerns against truthful harms from drinking alcohol, the government of Canada could casually continue collecting additional alcohol sales taxation revenues, worth windfall multi millions of extra dollars annually to Canada's federal treasury. Surprisingly, in less than fifteen years (by 1937) both the Canadian and U.S. federal governments were using similar methods of collecting alcohol sales taxation revenues from people, while publicly prohibiting and criticizing God's preferred green herb cannabis plants. By the fall of 1937, both the United States and Canadian federal governments enacted and rigorously enforced unusually severe and unfair public laws against nonharmful and constructive cannabis (marijuana) users, while eliminating public prohibition legislation against alcohol, a well known contributor to many miserable and true demonstrable harms, including deaths.

"The Canadian government stood to gain financially from smuggling operations. It levied a tax of $9.00 per gallon on alcohol consumed in Canada, but refunded this tax on liquor that had been exported, after presentation of a customs receipt from the country to which it was exported. Because smugglers could not furnish a receipt from United States customs officers, the tax remained with the Dominion government as if the alcohol really had been consumed at home, a bonus of $30 million a year, one fifth of all Dominion and provincial revenues."[414] Large volumes of alcohol faced few major obstacles moving from Canada into the United States during this time. "Professional smuggling from Canada was an easier business than smuggling from the open sea. It was close to large industrial cities such as Detroit, from which it was separated by short stretches of water. . . . At least 900,000 cases of liquor were transported within Canada to the border cities, in the first seven months of 1920. . . . Since customs offices were closed at night and

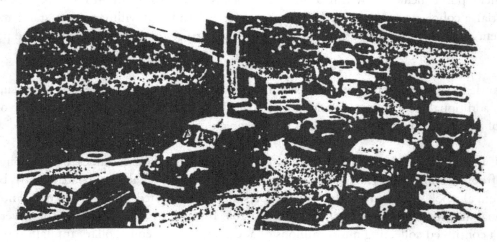

Footnote[415]

the border was largely unguarded, most smugglers made their journeys then. Caravans of as many as fourteen cars could pass unchallenged through the countryside around Lake Champlain."[416]

Near the mid 1920s, more complex and lucrative schemes were being used to smuggle large volumes of alcohol from Canada into the United States, with boats and railroad cars. "One device used by smugglers was to pretend to ship legal products from Buffalo to Detroit via Canada. The cars were inspected and sealed in Buffalo by customs officers. Liquor was substituted for the stated cargo in Canada, and then the cars with counterfeit seals were dispatched for Detroit, where they were not inspected a second time. Because of the capacity of railroad cars, the amounts of liquor smuggled in this way were huge as the few seizures indicate. On November 19, 1927 for instance, three railroad cars supposedly carrying gears were impounded at the North Detroit Station by prohibition agents, who discovered they contained $200,000 worth of whiskey and wine ready to be sold for Thanksgiving."[417] Ineffective enforcement procedures and incomplete plans culminated in many alcohol violations of and disregard for public prohibition laws against alcohol in the United States. J. Chapman reported in 'Outlook' on January 16, 1924 that alcohol prohibition was promoting three powerful popular passions: "the passion of the prohibitionists for law, the passion of the drinking classes for drink and the passion of the largest and best organized smuggling trade that has ever existed for money."[418]

In Canada during the early 1920s, governmental laws did not nationally prohibit alcohol drinking, transporting, importing or exporting, even though North American alcohol-involved violent crimes with severe harms began significantly increasing. Instead, with the Canadian federal legal system attention was diverted away from alcohol, a known producer of many violent truthful harms, and unfavourable attention began being directed against God's helpful green herb cannabis plants. This quiet political procedure would allow continuation of the lucrative annual multi-million dollar cash flow of additional alcohol taxation money into Canadian governments' treasuries.

Substantiated harms from alcohol violations in Canada continued increasing. "Convictions for drunken driving rose from 202 in 1922, to 1,322 in 1928. This was an increase of 554 percent in six years, during which time the numbers of cars on the roads only doubled."[419]

Regarding similar Canadian marijuana offences between 1922 and 1928 there were no actual recorded and truthfully-proven convictions of impaired driving due to personal ingestion of marijuana. Also, in relation to Canadian alcohol-produced demonstrable harms during this time span, "Statistics in Canada indicate that an increase in immoderate drinking . . . was partially responsible for an increase in serious crimes. In 1922, there were 15,720 convictions for indictable offences, and in 1928, 21,720 convictions, an increase of 38 percent and more than three times the increase in the population."[420]

Also, with alcohol-involved crimes between 1922 and 1928 in Canada, "the number of criminals who were immoderate drinkers increased by 64 percent."[421] During this same time, no official Canadian public reports show similar increases in actual criminals and violent crimes that were officially proven to be truthfully related to personal consumption of cannabis (marijuana). This compares with an actual sixty-four percent increase in the thousands of alcohol-drinking harm-producing violent criminals in Canada.

However, during this time a small group of influential people in the Canadian government and court system began publishing unsubstantiated and nonscientific statements against God's preferred and historically valuable green herb cannabis plants (marijuana). Within a few years, this secretive group of powerful public officials changed and enforced new Canadian legislation. For the first time in history, national laws were put into place making nonharmful public uses of God's preferred green herb cannabis plants a much more punishable criminal offence than public drinking of alcohol, God's worst enemy. In essence, discrimination and alcohol-drinking encouragement during the 1920s and 30s were significant reasons why unusual laws secretively emerged against God's helpful cannabis plants.

To build the first railroad across Canada, the Canadian government authorized importation of 17,000 Chinese labourers, of which more than 4,000 died in construction.[422] British merchants during this time had also been legally selling opium mainly to these Chinese labourers for easing, "the pain of their meager circumstances."[423] When the railroad had been built and the gold fields in B.C. and California exhausted, thousands of people found themselves seriously unemployed in Vancouver, British Columbia. With less work and more people, competition caused labour prices to generally decrease, thereby lowering living standards for all involved workers and their families. Instead of organizing more profitable production processes to keep everyone constructively employed, Mackenzie King decided to legally exclude or eliminate these Chinese workers from the Canadian labour market.[424] Then, remaining white workers could have higher wages. In 1907, Mackenzie King (federal Deputy Minister of Labour) visited Vancouver and noticed the unique legal practise of British merchants selling opium mostly to Chinese workers. To exclude or eliminate the Chinese from working in Canada, Mackenzie King drafted the Opium Narcotic Act of 1908. "In fact it is doubtful that Mackenzie King had ever intended the Act be applied to any segment of the white population at all."[425] Discrimination or racism was used to attempt increasing living standards for white people.

Eliminating competition from Chinese workers would mean higher wages for white workers, and deportation of these 'opium taking' Chinese workers.

Difficulties with enforcing the Opium Narcotic Act of 1908 and development of smuggling networks prompted official establishment of a Canadian Royal Commission on British and Chinese opium smuggling. Recommendations of this Commission resulted in authorization and enforcement of the Opium and Drug Act of 1911. For the first time in history, this Act expanded the list of prohibited drugs, while also making "simple use and possession of the prohibited drugs an offence, and widened police powers of search and seizure."[426]

In 1920, shortly before Mackenzie King became Prime Minister, the Opium and Drug Branch was established and put in charge of enforcing narcotics legislation. "The RCMP worked very closely with the Drug Branch and their service was rewarded with ever more lenient laws regarding their right to search and seize the property of suspected drug users."[427]

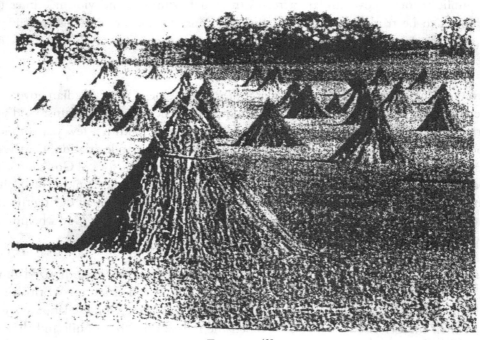

Footnote[428]

Emily Murphy, while residing in Edmonton, Alberta became Canada's first female police magistrate judge, and was also a leader of the Irish Orange Order an organized group, "which then wanted a pure white Canada."[429] This pro-discrimination attitude soon resulted in her writing and selling unsubstantiated and biased stories against God's green herb cannabis plants. Using the pretentious name of 'Janey Canuck', Emily Murphy, also a false-alarmist wrote and published a book, The Black Candle, which was, "very biased and sensationalized."[430] The RCMP used this book to increase its power, along with making cannabis (hemp) illegal, under its newly spelled legislated name, 'marijuana' in the Opium and Drug Act of 1923.[431] The quiet and official introduction of this strange new big word, 'marijuana' with a 'j' in the middle appeared in Canadian law dictionaries for the first time, truthfully meaning that a publicly popular and valuable medicinal plant, well-known as cannabis or hemp was now illegal, with no public input, debate or majority vote of approval. 'Marijuana' had previously been a Spanish word known to mean the cannabis or hemp plant. Without warning, God's medicinal cannabis plants suddenly became illegal for all Canadians to consume, with comparatively cruel and unusual punishments oppressively imposed for nonconformity. Freedom of individual choice was no longer legally available for trying to improve one's life, as with nonharmfully using helpful cannabis foods, clothes and medicines. Without public participation, Emily Murphy's legislation with Mackenzie King's authorization was imposed on Canadians, with no substantiated medical, scientific, moral or any other justified explanation. During this same discrimination era with democratic governments, three states in the U.S., similarly made cannabis illegal, "all without the benefit of any scientific studies."[432] As in Canada, "these laws were put into place to harass and deport minority groups."[433]

In 1922, Canadian judge Emily Murphy with nonscientific and unproven stories, "raised the alarm" of fear against God's green cannabis plants. Within a year, Canadian federal legislation imposed harmful punishments on people for nonharmfully using, possessing or growing God's green herb cannabis plants. Never before in North American history had cannabis/marijuana been placed under the legal man-made criminal category of 'narcotic'. Millions of alcohol taxation dollars could continue cascading into Canadian governments' coffers, by merely condemning marijuana for society's problems. Making big time easy money from alcohol taxation revenue was an ongoing priority. Also legalized was reducing penalties for alcohol related crimes, by giving leniencies to criminals if they said they were under the influence of alcohol when they did their harms. Protecting criminals instead of victims created an unjust society.

With this sudden and confusing man-made law, numerous innocent people soon became deprived of one of the earth's most helpful medicinal herb plants. In fact, in Canada marijuana was only unfairly suspected, but never proved to be an official public problem. Marijuana was not even presented as a proved problem, "in 1923 when it was first added to the schedule of prohibited 'narcotics'.

Similarly, it was still not assessed as a significant problem by a Special Committee in 1955."[434] Yet alcohol, known many times over as being involved with producing violent demonstrable harms continued to be legally available for public drinking, buying, selling, trafficking, importing and exporting. Also at this time, historically unusual punishments including arrests, monetary fines, searches and imprisonments suddenly began being enforced against people for cultivating, trafficking, selling, and/or personally using God's helpful green herb marijuana. Thousands of consecutive years of many

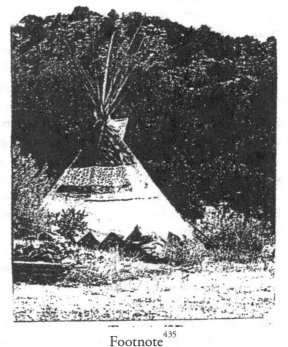

Footnote[435]

beneficial uses for: foods, clothing, shelters and medicines suddenly became disregarded by newly imposed man-made laws against helpful marijuana uses. Easy money, control, power, discrimination and alcohol were among the main reasons why marijuana suddenly became illegal.

About ten years after alcohol was publicly prohibited in the United States, the Canadian federal government decided to legally co-operate with U.S. governmental attempts at reducing alcohol-produced harms. In 1929, the Canadian federal government, under MacKenzie King, "introduced a bill in the House of Commons in Ottawa prohibiting the release of liquor for export to any country that had made it illegal to import beer, wine and spirits. . . . The bill became law on June 1, 1930."[436] Only limited exportation of products containing alcohol was prohibited in Canada at this time, not the manufacturing, importing, advertising, trafficking, selling, or drinking of alcohol.

In the United States between 1923 and 1937, official federal government sentiments, along with some news media of the time shifted focus, from condemning and reducing demonstrably harmful alcohol-drinking in America to promoting untrue and horrible fear stories against God's green herb marijuana.

A foremost promoter of such fictional fear fabrications from the U.S. was Harry Anslinger. "In 1929, Anslinger was still fighting a losing battle against alcohol."[437] This was when he obtained employment with the U.S. federal alcohol prohibition agency. Although, he publicly wrote false, alarmist and fear fostering stories that were not factually or truthfully supported, Anslinger still, "assumed control of the newly formed Bureau of Narcotics which was subsumed into the Treasury Department of the federal government, the concern over marijuana was just beginning to have a national impact."[438] It was near the end of the 1920s, the same time as when the New York stock market crashed, and slightly before the miserable depression of the 'dirty thirties'. In 1926, alarmist Harry Anslinger, "wrote an article exposing the myth that sharks attack humans, and revealed that it was in fact barracudas who are the culprits of the deep. Published in the June 12, 1926 issue of the Saturday Evening Post, Anslinger debunked the shark's bad image with, "It may be safely stated that unless a shark is ravenously hungry he will not attack a human being, unless he is positive that the man has been drowned or is absolutely helpless. It has never been known to attack anything that is perfectly healthy. It didn't take long for a torrent of letters to swamp the magazine's desks. People from all over the world sent in protesting letters documenting horrible experiences where sharks had attacked healthy humans. . . . Australians regard with astonishment persons who claim that the vicious barracuda is responsible for attacks by sharks. They have many arguments to back up their claim that the shark is a man-eater. Early in 1927, a fifteen-year-old boy died as a result of being attacked by a shark at Port Hacking, Australia. . . . It was found that the flesh of the right leg had been torn completely off, from the thigh to the ankle leaving the bones exposed and causing death shortly thereafter. . . .

In the summer of 1926, a shark captured at Koolau, Hawaii was found to contain human bones and a pair of swimming trunks. The bones consisted of more than half of the upper part of a skull, a hand, a knee, and two whole arms."[439] Harry Anslinger publicly described false and unsubstantiated fear fostering stories about killing and eating practices of sharks, considering himself to be an authority on the subject. Perhaps, he similarly concluded that alcohol didn't produce demonstrable harms to people either, contrary to an abundance of substantiated facts and truths existing before and at this time.

During the 1920s, Harry Anslinger was an employee of the U.S. federal alcohol prohibition agency responsible for enforcing the National Prohibition Act, also known as the Volstead Act. A primary purpose of this alcohol prohibition agency was to prohibit, or at least noticeably reduce amounts of alcohol being drank by people in the United States. The continuous obvious ineffectiveness of operations conducted by Harry Anslinger and his agents, in reducing and eliminating the drinking of alcohol by people in the U.S., soon became evident. Actual proof and substantiation of this was publicly known. Reliable reports began being published, such as the following. "It is clear however, that liquor was being sold all over New York, and that the number of places where it was available ran well into the tens of thousands. During the mid 1920s, complaints of Volstead Act violations were being referred to federal authorities by the police, at a rate of fifteen thousand a month.

The best answer to the question of where the speakeasies could be found was given by the New York Telegram which said in 1929:

Where on Manhattan Island can you buy liquor?

Answer: In open saloons, restaurants, night clubs, bars behind a peephole, dancing academies, drugstores, delicatessens, cigar stores, confectioneries, soda fountains, behind partitions of shoeshine parlours, back rooms of barbershops, from hotel bellhops, from hotel headwaiters, from hotel day clerks, night clerks, in express offices, in motorcycle delivery agencies, paint stores, malt shops, cider stubes, fruit stands, vegetable markets, taxi drivers, grocery shops, smoke shops, athletic clubs, grillrooms, taverns, chophouses, importing firms, tearooms, moving-van companies, spaghetti houses, boarding-houses, Republican clubs, Democratic clubs, laundries, social clubs, and newspapermen's associations."[440] Harry Anslinger and the agency in which he was employed simply did not effectively cope with several large and sometimes gaping loopholes in enforcement practises of alcohol prohibition in the United States.

Another place where illegal drinking of alcohol and serious demonstrable harms were occurring in America, during this time was in 'clip joints'. The following report from the mid 1920s describes related conditions about additional ineffective enforcement practices of alcohol prohibition laws in the United States. "One of the most profitable branches of the nightclub business was the 'clip joint' which for downright viciousness was equalled only by the worst of the old-time saloons. These fragrant dives were usually hidden away in a side street. . . . The typical clip joint was staffed by a bartender, two or three waiters who doubled as strong-arm men, a tough floor manager, a singer and piano player, a half-naked cigarette girl, and from two to ten hostesses, depending upon the size of the place. The sucker was usually brought to the clip joint by a taxi driver, or sent there by a hotel clerk. He was assured that he would find girls galore and lots of good liquor, "right off the boat."

When he arrived, he was immediately importuned to buy drinks for one or more of the hostesses who intimated they would be available for more interesting activities, "after we get through work." The girls usually drank 'gin highballs' which were compounded of water and a little orange juice or ginger ale, and for which the sucker was charged from one to two dollars. The sucker himself for his initial drink was given a double slug of raw alcohol doctored to resemble whiskey. If he got helplessly drunk, he was simply robbed and dumped into the gutter a block or so away from the clip joint. If, through some miracle he remained fairly sober and showed a disposition to quit spending, the usual procedure was for one of the hostesses to accuse him of insulting her. Thereupon, the floor manager would indignantly tell him to leave and present him with a bill, an outrageous compilation which included: a large cover charge, a dozen drinks he hadn't ordered, all those he had already paid for, a bottle or two of liquor, a half dozen packs of cigarettes at a dollar each, and extras. If he paid, he was permitted to depart, although he was lucky if a sympathetic hostess didn't pick his pocket before he reached the door. If he protested, he was kicked and slugged until he was groggy or unconscious, after which he was robbed and thrown out. The police seldom raided a politically protected night club."[441] Public drinking of prohibited alcohol in America was far more rampant than initial legislation intended. Lack of effective enforcement, and many individual opportunities for amassing additional illegal financial wealth, along with quests for power and control contributed to disintegration and dissolvement of the U.S. national alcohol prohibition legislation.

Actual politics of the day also began interfering with intended successes of alcohol prohibition laws in the United States during the late 1920s. For example, with the U.S. presidential election campaign of 1928, the Democratic Party (the 'wets') nominated New York's Governor Alfred E. Smith. Many alcohol prohibitionists opposed him, "primarily because he was a wet."[442] Again, 'wets' were people who personally drank alcohol or supported the practise of other people drinking alcohol.

Nearly four years later, in the U.S. presidential election campaign of 1932, the Democratic Party led by Franklin D. Roosevelt adopted a platform to repeal or abolish laws that prohibited manufacturing or selling alcohol. Many federal politicians of the day began promoting the notion of legally allowing the public to drink alcohol. After all, this was supposed to be a free country and a democracy heralded as, 'The Land of the Free' in its own national anthem. Legal changes soon occurred, "amid great disorder with boos and hisses for the few dry delegates who tried to protest. The plank said, "We favor repeal of the Eighteenth Amendment" and demanded that Congress immediately submit a repeal amendment to state conventions. . . . What most of the voters seem to remember however was what Franklin Roosevelt said when he made his dramatic appearance at the Democratic convention to accept the U.S. presidential nomination. "I say to you," he shouted, "that from this date on the Eighteenth Amendment is doomed!"[443] Little did he realize his own country and many other areas of the world would soon be doomed to blatantly harmful realities of: depressions, droughts, hungers, poverties, miseries, pains, wars, injuries, casualties, despairs and deaths.

President Roosevelt's own name would soon be added to the grim reaper's list of dead liquor drinking promoters, as related alcohol taxation revenues kept topping up government coffers.

During the late 1920s and early 'dirty-thirties' U.S. public opinion leaned in the direction of having man-made laws allowing people to drink alcohol a known producer of numerous violent demonstrable harms. "The consequent identification of wet and dry with specific political parties meant the Democratic victory in the 1930 congressional elections was identified as one favoring the wet cause . . . and the Democratic victory in 1932 was thus considered a mandate for repeal of the 18th Amendment."[444] On a cold and windy February day in 1933, the U.S. Federal House and Senate adopted a resolution proposing the 21st Amendment to the United States Constitution, thereby repealing the Eighteenth Amendment of the U.S. Constitution. Finally, on a frigid December 5th in 1933 the official amendment and repeal of public alcohol prohibition laws was authorized with man-made legislation.[445] Government liquor taxation revenues would flow in faster than ever before as harm-producing alcohol once again became legal for millions of people to drink, amid a very dangerous atmosphere.

Meantime, legal federal attention in the United States without conclusive factual and truthful substantiation soon moved in the direction of blaming God's green herb marijuana plants for producing public harms. In the U.S. federal government on August 12, 1930, the Federal Bureau of Narcotics (FBN) became legally established, "under the aegis of the Treasury Department, with Harry Anslinger appointed as the FBN's first Commissioner."[447] Anslinger would be the one and only Commissioner of this newly formed Federal Bureau of Narcotics, for more than thirty consecutive years until 1962. By the mid 1930s, inaccurate shark story teller and operationally ineffective federal alcohol prohibition enforcement employee, Harry Anslinger conducted a leading role in the man-made legal push prohibiting people from using marijuana plants. Although, God's preferred green herb cannabis plants were known throughout history as truthfully having many constructive and helpful attributes, including producing beneficial medicines, foods, clothes and shelters, irrespectively Harry Anslinger and related influential secretive federal government officials, including Andrew Mellon and Herman Oliphant contrived and conducted an American legal campaign against God's natural cannabis plants. Other involved industrialists included: the Duponts (plastics, petrochemicals and vehicles), the Rockerfellars (petroleum products), and the Hearsts (national newspaper fabricated sensationalism).

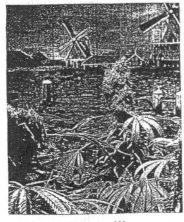

Footnote[446]

Harry Anslinger's father-in-law of all people was Andrew Mellon, who at this time occupied the powerful position of Secretary of the U.S. Federal Treasury Department. It is interesting to observe that at and after this time Andrew Mellon was regarded as being the richest man in America. It also became known that Andrew Mellon was the wealthy and powerful owner of Gulf Oil.[448] Furthermore, it was Andrew Mellon and his secretive Treasury Department who, "pushed legislation through Congress giving tax breaks to oil companies."[449] In addition, it was Andrew Mellon who, "lent Du Pont money to purchase General Motors."[450] General Motors then went on to become the largest company in North America.

Another significantly involved and secretive U.S. federal employee was Herman Oliphant, who became Chief Counsel of the U.S. Treasury Department during the mid 1930s and beyond. Of course Andrew Mellon was Herman Oliphant's boss. At the same time, Andrew Mellon was also Harry Anslinger's boss and father-in-law.

It became quietly known that Harry Anslinger, "was nephew-in-law to Secretary of the Treasury, Andrew Mellon a banker who was financing the growing petrochemical dynasty of the Du Ponts. Mellon had designed Anslinger's position personally."[451] This closely knit, secretive and powerful group of people created and implemented a set of legal plans, that would no longer allow public benefits from God's green herb marijuana plants. Never before in U.S. history had this ever happened.

"The petrochemical and pulp-paper industries in particular stood to lose billions of dollars, if the commercial potential of hemp was fully realized. Researcher Jack Herer names Hearst and Du Pont as two of the interests most responsible for orchestrating the demise of hemp manufacturing.

In the 1920s, the Du Pont company developed and patented fuel additives such as tetraethyl lead, as well as the sulphate and sulphite processes for manufacture of pulp, paper and numerous synthetic products such as nylon, cellophane and other plastics."[452]

It also happened that a modern machine had been recently invented, successfully tested, and was about to be mass produced with assembly-line technology. This new efficient machine, capable of vastly increasing marijuana plant harvesting, in terms of improved output quality, quantity and timing received the commercial name of hemp decorticator.[453] Fast and effective marijuana processing machines, their assembly-line production, along with marijuana biomass fuels, and marijuana plastics developments would allow huge tracts of timberland to continue producing abundant amounts of healthy oxygen for the nation. However, such a healthy course of public democratic action would probably, "eliminate much of the need for wood-pulp paper, thus threatening to drastically reduce values of the vast timber-lands still owned by Hearst."[454]

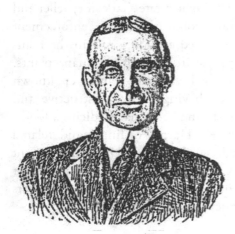

Footnote[455]

Henry Ford and other constructive producers began encouraging a more environmentally friendly approach to vehicle engine emissions. They, "were developing synthetic products from renewable biomass resources, especially hemp."[456] It soon became known that, "Ford and other companies were already promising to make every product from cannabis carbohydrates that was currently being made from petroleum hydrocarbons."[457] It is recorded, "by the 1930s the Ford Motor Company was creating charcoal fuel, creosote, ethyl-acetate, methanol and other compounds out of hemp, at their . . . biomass conversion plant at Iron Mountain, Michigan. Ford envisioned a future where plastics from hemp polymers were the building blocks of almost all products, and where fuel was provided by hemp biomass, and he gave the world a glimpse of that future with his all-organic car. Mechanical Engineering magazine heralded

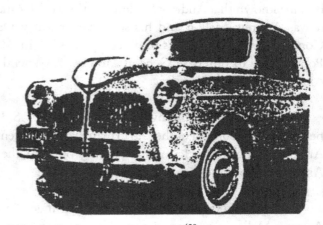

Footnote[458]

hemp, in its February 1937 issue as, "the most profitable and desirable crop that can be grown."[459] It is also recorded that Henry Ford, "grew marijuana on his estate after 1937. He even made plastic cars with wheat straw, hemp and sisal."[460]

Among the secretive political actions in the U.S., "from 1935 to 1937 Du Pont lobbied the Chief Counsel of the Treasury Department, Herman Oliphant for prohibition of cannabis, assuring him that DuPont's synthetic petrochemicals (such as urethane) could replace hemp-seed oil in the market place.

Some large pharmaceutical companies also stood to gain with illegalization of cannabis, since their synthetic patented prescription transquillizers (such as barbiturates) would find room in the void left by prohibition of this natural relaxant."[461]

In addition, during 1935-1937 the very influential and secretive cluster of: Mellon, Du Pont, Hearst, Oliphant and Anslinger began seriously condemning God's traditionally helpful green herb marijuana plants. Hearst and Anslinger promoted publicly printing and publishing sensentionalized fabricated fear stories against God's green herb marijuana, but presenting such fearful fictional fabrications as though they were true, in essence fearfully misleading the public. Anslinger had previous public fear-fostering experience as with his false alarming shark stories of the 1920s. From 1933 to 1937, U.S. federal government's man-made laws and policies promoted harm-producing alcohol-drinking for society, while condemning, restricting and legally prohibiting God's helpful green herb marijuana plants. This was when Andrew Mellon's secretive U.S. Treasury staff formed a new legal word, by removing the 'j' from marijuana (as recently legally created in Canada) and replacing it with an 'h' spelling a new legal word, 'marihuana' with an 'h' in the middle. The U.S. public had never seen this big unusual legal word before. But this new word, marihuana would soon become nationally illegal, with comparatively cruel and unusual punishments forcefully imposed for nonconformity. Some influential governmental officials then began blaming society's violent demonstrable harms on this new word with an 'h' in the middle, instead of the real truth that the government had recently re-legalized public alcohol-drinking throughout the country for the first time in over a decade.

Suddenly however, during the mid 1930s many new, untrue, shocking, unsubstantiated, horrible and fearful newspaper fiction stories were being sold to the public, as though such fabrications were true. One such unsubstantiated and widely distributed newspaper story exclaims, "Shocking crimes of violence are increasing. Murders, slaughterings . . . authorities attribute much of this violence to . . . marihuana."[462] Blaming this new word, with an 'h' in the middle meant more taxed alcohol could be made available for the public to drink. While government coffers swelled with more tax cash, related harms could then be blamed on God's green herb marijuana plants. Who could argue with a strange official word they had never seen before, especially dispersed from a senior U.S. government office? In truthful reality, this new legal word really meant the hemp (cannabis) plant known to have been successfully commercially cultivated for thousands of years, as a leading natural resource in many countries throughout the world. Millions of farmers would soon be harmfully treated by being legally forced out of work, along with having miseries of poverty and depression, while also being legally forced to consume less nutritious and medically inferior foods and medicines. Harms against humanity are crimes against humanity.

Rather than concluding significant legislative changes allowing increased legal public access to drinking alcohol truthfully contributed to increased violent harms, some influential officials chose instead to blame God's green herb marihuana plants. Such untrue and unjust actions were soon

By: Joseph W. Jacob B.A., M.P.A.

officially occuring in the U.S., without regard for democratic, traditional, scientific or medically substantiated evidence.

Harry Anslinger, one of these influential officials did not have an abundance of actual agricultural experience and specialized education required to be correctly classified as an horticultural authority specializing in uses and knowledge of natural green herb hemp (marihuana) plants. Anslinger was more used to journals, ledgers, taxes, account numbers, false fear stories, and imposing additional arbitrary laws including unusually severe and unjustified punishments against many nonharmful citizens in a 'free-country' with a constitutional democracy.

Surprisingly, violent demonstrably harmful and specific characteristics previously well known about people drinking alcohol were now being publicly, fictitiously and shockingly applied against God's medically helpful marihuana plants.

This new and untruthful attitude soon spread throughout many harmful elements of society, and criminals were soon receiving judges' leniencies and abstinences from punishments for their true harms if such criminals merely said marihuana caused their crimes. In the mid 1930s, an official U.S. federal report concludes, "We have reliable information that the word is being passed along through the young underworld to 'blame it on the weed' when tried for a crime."[463] (Weed was commonly known to mean marihuana, cannabis or hemp.)

Man-made laws against God's natural and preferred marihuana plants were soon being contrived and pushed by a small self serving cluster of secretive influential officials within the U.S. federal government. "In the secret Treasury Department meetings conducted between 1935 and 1937 prohibitive tax laws were drafted and strategies plotted."[464]

The Marihuana Tax Act of 1937 quickly ended traditional legal large scale marihuana farming in America, in addition to medium and small scale farming or cultivating God's favoured green herb marijuana plants. When the Federal Bureau of Narcotics secretively ushered this tax bill (not a health bill) through the U.S. federal government (without usual democratic debates, truths and votes) it immediately

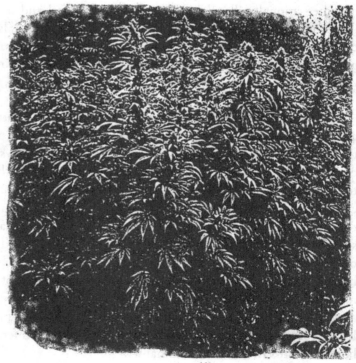

Footnote[465]

became financially prohibitive for American farmers to continue cultivating hemp plants. The small, influential and secretive U.S. Treasury Department, "pushed through Congress a bill taxing hemp

86

at the rate of $1.00 per ounce for industrial and medical purposes, and $100.00 per ounce for other purposes."[466] No profit-minded farmer could afford to continue cultivating and harvesting marihuana plants with these unprecedented excessive tax rates. This economically and medically cruel and unusual legislation was similar to imposing an extra tax of $1.00 an ounce on wheat, corn or potatoes. When farmers were only receiving less than a dollar per bushel (e.g. 25 lbs.) for traditional agricultural products, how could they afford to pay an extra tax of about four hundred dollars per bushel? ($1.00 per ounce, times 16 ounces per pound, times 25 pounds per bushel is $400.) And the extra marihuana tax became one hundred times this amount (or $40,000 (that is: forty thousand dollars per bushel) if it was to be used for purposes other than commercial or medical. How could any farmer, or any other rational person afford to pay an extra confusing tax of between four hundred and forty thousand dollars per bushel, when these farmers were only receiving less than a dollar per bushel for selling marijuana plants, or corn, or wheat or potatos? This unusually severe, man-made and secretively contrived 'first time' U.S. marihuana tax law cruelly harmed and economically decimated a constructive public agricultural industry, by throwing at least millions of people out of work, while depriving American's free enterprise democracy of at least millions of dollars worth of beneficial medicines and foods known to have helped improve and sustain peoples' lives. This is inconsistent with guaranteed constitutional rights and freedoms advocating life and liberty in both official constitutions of Canada and the United States. An unjust society emerged.

The secretive details and actual papers for approval were formed in Andrew Mellon's and Harry Anslinger's U.S. Treasury Department. All that remained was having another senior official in the U.S. Treasury Department, Herman Oliphant casually arrange to bypass the usual official democratic debate process in the U.S. Congress with this new tax bill, and have it directly and immediately approved by the U.S. Government's 'Ways and Means Committee'.

Near the middle of April 1937, "Herman Oliphant made his move. On April 14, 1937 he introduced the bill directly to the House Ways and Means Committee, instead of other appropriate committees such as Food and Drug, Agriculture, Textiles, Commerce, etc.

The reason may have been that the Ways and Means is the only committee to send its bills directly to the House floor, without the act having to be debated upon by other committees.

Ways and Means Chairman Robert L. Doughton . . . quickly rubber-stamped the secret Treasury bill and sent it sailing through Congress to the President."[467]

Dr. James Woodward, who was both a physician and an attorney at this time was not pleased with the secretive and unusual legislative procedures used, including disregard of medical advice from the American Medical Association (AMA). "We cannot understand yet, Mr. Chairman, why this bill should have been prepared in secret for two years, without any intimation even to the profession protested Woodward, that it was being prepared."[468] Despite reliable testimony to the contrary, based on true and factual medical, scientific and practical evidence, the Marihuana Tax Act nevertheless became strictly enforced in the United States beginning on the first day of September 1937, as traffic in marihuana became federally prohibited. In the US., this was the, "first federal legislation prohibiting the unregulated traffic in marihuana."[469] Secretive selfish laws *not* intended to be *for* the people or by the people reduced national nutritional and prosperity standards. Miseries not happiness were on the dark, dismal and dangerous horizon.

An act involving taxation, with not even any mention of health or morality issues, legally prohibited people from nonharmfully medically using marihuana. Taxes, secrecy, discrimination, power and control were relevant reasons why marihuana was legally banned from constructive public uses in America. Respected and well-informed medical people protested, but to no avail. During 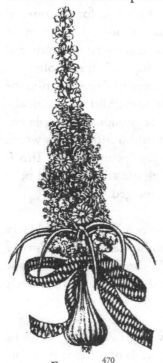 1937, members of the Committee on Legislative Activities of the American Medical Association wrote and submitted letters officially protesting the proposed U.S. federal Marihuana Tax Act. Among, the logical, medical and other beneficial reasons presented for marihuana's continued public uses is an official medical statement concluding, "There is positively no evidence to indicate the abuse of cannabis as a medicinal agent. . . . It would seem worthwhile to maintain its status as a medicinal agent for such purposes as it now has."[471] These reputable and humane medical recommendations, however were sidetracked from public democratic debate, by some influential secretive federal government officials. Prohibition of marihuana became hastily enforced in America, without even having a public debate or democratic vote (referendum) on this new important law, that would demonstrably harm millions of democratic citizens, by depriving them of traditionally helpful, life-promoting vitamins, nutrients, medicines and foods, in addition to their usual jobs and livelihoods. A demonstrably harmful world-wide depression, including a major stock market crash, dirty-thirties and gruesome global war lurked dangerously ahead.

Footnote[470]

Abraham Lincoln, when democratically speaking 'for' the people, by the people and of the people typically promoted the concept of the greatest good for the greatest number of people. Abraham Lincoln truthfully spoke out against prohibition. As President Lincoln explains, "Prohibition . . . goes beyond the bounds of reason, in that it attempts to control a man's appetite by legislation, and makes a crime out of things that are not crimes. . . . A prohibition law strikes a blow at the very principles upon which our government was founded."[472] Principles of governments 'for' the people, majority-vote rule, equal benefit of the law, actions adding value without harm, as well as advocating life, liberty and happiness are among the basic democratic principles referred to by honest Abraham Lincoln.

Why were taxation bureaucrats given unusual responsibilities relating to peoples' health? A U.S. federal health department was in existence at, and before this time. A report to the United States Congress, from the U.S. Department of Health, Education and Welfare advises, "Until 1937, marihuana in some form was a staple in many U.S. patent medicines. . . . Nevertheless, there were 28 pharmaceutical preparations containing cannabis in use, when passage of the Marihuana Tax Act in 1937 banned cannabis as a medicine."[473] Many valuable, trusted and helpful medical uses of marihuana had been developed and successfully used by the public. Marihuana was, "being prescribed for sedation, senile insomnia, menstrual disorders, epilepsy, severe neuralgia and migraine."[474] In addition, marijuana cigarettes had been legally marketed for many consecutive years as, "a remedy for asthma."[475]

Between 1850 and 1937 marihuana, "was used as the prime medicine for more than 100 separate illnesses or diseases, in the U.S. pharmacopoeia."[476] One legal over-the-counter marihuana remedy, from the Eli Lilly company was named the, 'One Day Cough Cure'.[477] A moderate amount of marihuana leaves and/or seed goods were likely swallowed, followed by drinking teas of marihuana leaves, and smoking pleasant smelling buds and/or resins of marihuana plants. Relaxation and expectoration for removing unwanted phlegm would likely then result in the cough not being bothersome within a day or so.

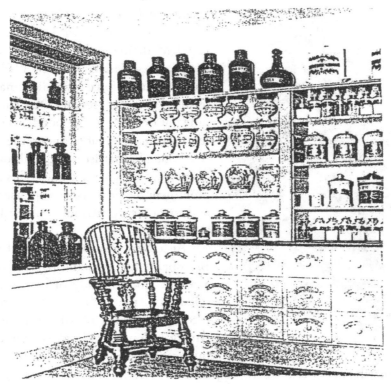

Footnote[478]

Marihuana plant goods were also being popularly used for manufacturing clothing. For example, "Before 1937 Levi jeans were made of hemp."[479] Such beneficial and nonharmful uses however were irrationally ignored by some influential U.S. federal personnel involved, including Harry Anslinger, Herman Oliphant and their boss Andrew Mellon.

It's interesting and true that rich Andrew Mellon, whose man-made laws deprived America of helpful medicines, foods and clothing, while causing unprecedented harmful public unemployment, lost his life just a few days before marihuana prohibition laws officially began in the U.S. Andrew Mellon suddenly died on August 27, 1937. A close associate of his Mr. Pope died the next night. Ogden Mills and Parker Gilbert both devoted friends of Andrew Mellon drove to Mellon's funeral together, "and both of these men died within the year."[480]

In the United States, federal narcotic laws began being regulated with the Harrison Act of 1914. For a short while in the U.S., cannabis, "was included in the early drafts of that legislation, however due to vocal opposition of the pharmaceutical and medical professions, it was later dropped."[481] Humane and logical reasons in 1914, by respected officials of the American medical profession (a related public authority) provided honest leadership in maintaining a legal and logical distinction between marihuana and other different products known to have caused many miserable harms to people, real and true narcotics, such as heroin, alcohol and codeine. Only true narcotics produce proven harms to peoples' bodies.

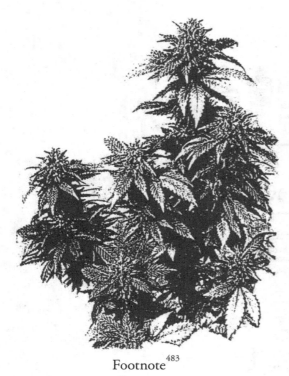

Footnote[483]

"One of the people to whom Anslinger addressed a series of fundamental questions about cannabis was William Woodward, Director of the Bureau of Legal Medicine and Legislation of the American Medical Association. The AMA, who by 1930 was a potent political force in medical matters had uneasy relations with the Treasury Department. . . . Twenty-nine out of the thirty respondents objected strongly to including cannabis under the Narcotic Drugs Act. One pharmacist railed, "Absolute rot. It is not necessary. I have never known of its misuse."[482] Other prominent medical people expressed similar positive and encouraging attributes of marihuana.

At a New York City hospital in 1934, Walter Bromberg, an assistant psychiatrist reported on a recent clinical study of marihuana, the specific scientific facts, observations, conclusions and recommendations of which were printed in the American Journal of Psychiatry, a respected medical publication. Bromberg, while presenting the first scientific data on marihuana since the fictional public scare stories of the early dirty-thirties concluded marihuana itself, "was not primarily responsible for crime. . . . Bromberg reported that not a single case of confirmed marihuana addiction was found in a group of 2,216 criminals convicted of felonies, in the Court of General Sessions in New York in 1933. "None of the assault crimes could be said to have been committed under the drug's influence."[484] Alcohol, meantime was significantly involved in producing at least hundreds of thousands of true, substantiated and violent demonstrable harms in America.

Another objective report, about man-made legal changes against marihuana users in the U.S. concludes, "The 1937 legislation was passed by Congress, largely at the behest of the Federal Bureau of Narcotics, without any genuine inquiry into the facts."[485] No truthfully substantiated health harms, or true moral reasons were officially provided or explained, regarding why marihuana suddenly became prohibited and criminalized by man-made laws and punishments in democratic America.

When the Marihuana Tax Act was passed in 1937, God's green herb marihuana suddenly and without just cause received the illegal classification of 'narcotic'. But, 'nowhere . . . in the committee hearings, or in the Congressional Record was there any discussion of the rationale for the drug classification."[486] Man-made laws, harmfully affecting health, life, liberty and happiness concerns for millions of people, in a democratic country were written, approved and officially enforced, "without any genuine inquiry into the facts" and without, "any discussion of the rationale." Such arbitrary actions harmfully affected lives for millions of Americans, many of whom probably regarded such severe and hurtful actions as cruel and unusual treatment. Quickly responding to behestful requests from Harry Anslinger (the 'shark-false-alarmist') and his Treasury Department took precedence over democratically improving living standards with objective, reliable, truthful, scientific, medical, moral, traditional and logical observations and conclusions. In a democratic country, important national health matters of a 'significant-change-nature' should be decided by at least the majority of the people in the country, not merely a minority of alarmist-oriented selfish public servants from non-health departments, as with Andrew Mellon, Harry Anslinger and Herman Oliphant. Government for the people, by the people, and of the people are prominent principles of free enterprise democratic justice, along with equal benefit of the law, and consistently providing the truth, the whole truth, and nothing but the truth, so help us God.

Even Harry Anslinger finally admitted his lack of evidence about truthfully relating causes of harmful crimes to marihuana. "On December 23, 1936 responding to an inquiry about crime and marihuana from P.F. Collier and Son magazine publishers, Anslinger was forced to admit that the Bureau's data was suspect:

So far as I know, no student of crime has as yet made any direct study of the relative percentage of violent crime which is attributable to the use of marihuana. [He obviously was not yet aware of Bromberg, or had forgotten]"[487] Although, Harry Anslinger had no related substantiated scientific evidence and truthfully proven facts, as well as non specialized and extensive personal education about marihuana plants, he nevertheless was directly involved with legally prohibiting millions of people in a democratic society from constructively using God's favoured, healthful and trusted marihuana plants.

When Harry Anslinger was asked for truthful and specific information relating marihuana to actual demonstrable harms, he was unable to provide proven evidence, neither with scientific nor with medical or moral facts. A response stated, "no one has been produced from the Bureau of Prisons to show the number of prisoners who have been found addicted to the marihuana habit. An informal inquiry shows that the Bureau of Prisons has no evidence on that point."[488] Millions of valuable lives became cruelly and unusually harmed by an informal inquiry.

"In fact, F.B.I. statistics had Anslinger bothered to check, showed at least 65% to 75% of all murders in the U.S. were then—and still are alcohol-related."[489]

Despite its incomplete understanding of truthful knowledge about natural green herb marihuana plants, the man-made, "Federal Bureau of Narcotics decisively shaped public discussion and the law for over two-and-a-half decades."[490] Here, in a prominent democratic society the majority of its participants were not included in actually making ongoing important decisions affecting their health, life, liberty and happiness standards. No specific public national referendum was ever officially conducted authorizing ongoing prohibition of green herb marihuana plants in North America. Instead, a small secretive group of selfish officials had controlling influence in planning, designing, approving and enforcing new man-made marihuana laws. This secretive legislation contributed to decreased health and living standards for millions of people in a free-enterprise democracy, whose purposes are to promote life, liberty, and happiness. Lost medical values alone were immense, as everyone could no longer legally use medicines from these helpful, multi-useful and traditionally trusted plants.

Next, comparatively cruel and unusual punishments were soon being enforced for not complying with these new man-made laws. Usually, responsible democratic justice is premised on equating the severity of the punishment to the severity of the crime or the truthful harm done, thereby balancing the scales of fundamental justice, using the truth, the whole truth and nothing but the truth, so help us God. However, with American marihuana legislation, this was not done. On August 2, 1937, Franklin D. Roosevelt signed the Marihuana Tax Act, "effectively making the use and sale of marihuana federal offences."[491] An unprecedented and unjustified cruel and unusual punishment schedule soon became publicly enforced for a hypothetical crime with no truthfully proven harm(s) produced by it. "Punishment on the federal level for violation of the Act may result in maximum sentences of from ten to forty years, depending on the offence if one possesses, sells, or gives away cannabis, without filling in the prescribed federal form."[492] Instead of applying the traditional legal democratic principle of equating the actual value of truthful harm produced with the actual value of punishment imposed, unexpected cruel and unusual punishments instead were described and enforced, where no truthfully substantiated harm was being produced by the nonharmful people being punished. The apparent harmful crime was not filling in a newly described, secretively-contrived, difficult-to-obtain, man-made, governmental paper form, from a small and confusing Treasury Department known for its nepotism and favouritism.

In the developing democracy of Canada, a similar arbitrary imposition occurred against constructive and nonharmful users of God's helpful green herb marijuana plants, again with no specific and truthful national referendum or plebiscite ever having been voted on and approved by the Canadian public. "Unauthorized cannabis cultivation was legally prohibited in 1938."[493] Although, these man-made laws apply to the Canadian public in a democracy whose anthem proclaims Canada to be 'Glorious and Free' the general Canadian public has never been included in any official specific democratic provincial or national majority-vote referendum authorizing these harmfully cruel, unusual and oppressive marijuana laws.

Between 1920 and 1937, North America legalized alcohol (God's worst enemy) and publicly prohibited using God's approved and preferred marijuana plants. The country then stumbled into an economic mess of troubles and tragedies: the stock market crashed in 1929, then came the great depression with forced legal closure of one of North America's largest agricultural industries (hemp/ marihuana), then came the dirty-thirties, quickly followed with world-wide fighting, harming and killing during destructive and disastrous World War Two.

But, there remained some peaceful people in the South Pacific, who preferred ingesting marijuana, as compared to drinking alcohol. To paraphrase a Rastafarian poet:

There Is No Comparison Between Marijuana And Alcohol

The Former Makes You 'Cool' The Latter Makes You Fall

Alcohol As We Know Is An Agent Of Death

With Using Marijuana You Draw New Breath[494]

Serious religious Rastafarian people maintain that marijuana ingestion, "induces wisdom and understanding and assists in reasoning, meditating, praying and communicating."[495] Marijuana ingestion, "produces a clarity of vision and depth of comprehension about man and his world, which is not attainable otherwise."[496] Marijuana, "is really used to bring forth a peaceful and complacent aspect within man."[497]

In less than twenty years of relatively recent history, immense amounts of truthful and demonstrable harms seriously afflicted North American citizens and the rest of the world, who were designing, imposing and enforcing similar man-made laws and punishments against nonharmful marijuana users. Alcohol, distrust, unemployment, poverty, marijuana-medicine-prohibition, depression, drought, fighting, shooting, killing, pain, sorrow, anguish, despair, and many other demonstrable harms resulted, as factual and true characteristics of this cruel, unusual, dangerous, disrespectful, secretive and arbitrary time frame. Less than twenty (20) years of recent history cruelly, unusally and harmfully changed at least ten thousand previous years of recorded history, in relation to people publicly and legally consuming God's helpful, natural and preferred green herb marijuana plants, in a variety of beneficial and nonharmful ways.

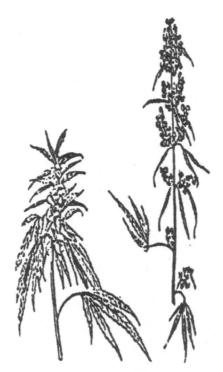

Footnote[498]

CHAPTER FIVE

CURRENT LAWS PREVENT MEDICAL BENEFITS

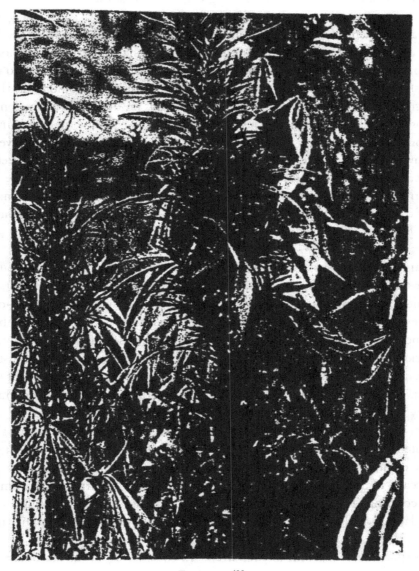

Footnote[499]

Unemployment, poverty, hunger, misery, desperation, threats, aggressions, guns, bullets, battles, bombs, war clouds, obliterations, deaths and graveyards horrified the world, within two years of 'alcohol-allowed and marijuana-prohibited' man-made laws in North America. The year 1939 marked the first year of gruesome World War Two, the largest military confrontation in history. Andrew Mellon, Harry Anslinger, Herman Oliphant and Adolf Hitler were contemporary influential public policy makers, whose actions harmfully affected lives of at least millions of people around the world. In January 1939, Harry Anslinger testified about his proposed 1940 bureau budget. "Again, marihuana was the Commissioner's whipping boy and this time he stressed the large eradication program the Bureau had undertaken."[500] This harmful, hypocritical, unsubstantiated, fear-filled approach repeated itself over and over, during the dirty-thirties, the destructive forties and into the continuing alcohol and pollution era of the fifties, the sixties and beyond. During this time era of depravations and true harms, "the United States Federal Bureau of Narcotics, under the direction of Commissioner H. Anslinger conducted a campaign against cannabis."[501]

An important element of fundamental justice was never evident with Mellon, Anslinger and their Treasury department's campaign against natural green herb marihuana plants, namely that punishments for proven demonstrable harms produced should always be equated to the severity of truthful harm(s) actually produced. Or, the severity of the punishment should always be equal to the severity of the crime. If low or no truthful and proven harm is produced, then low or no punishment should be imposed. Scales of fundamental justice are intended to equate actual punishments imposed to actual previous harms produced. This basic principle of fundamental justice, however has not been applied to many people who have used, sold, or transported marihuana with no related personal harm(s) produced in North America since 1937. "It is further considered that the legislation, in relation to marihuana was ill-advised, that it branded as a menace and crime a matter of trivial importance."[502] These new laws, however soon began delivering death to people who had not harmed anyone.

When discussing the unusual disproportionate severity of harmful government punishments for transporting or trafficking marihuana plants, Harry Anslinger describes an understanding he had with some farmers in Minnesota. "I will say that the farmers up there have been co-operating with us 100%. If they see anybody around that section who looks like a trafficker, they bring out their old shotguns and he is soon disposed of."[503] These violently harmful actions were extremely unfair. For mere suspicion, people were disposed of by shotgun blasts, without democratic justice including: truthfully proven harm(s) produced, due process of law, and equating the punishment to the truthful harm produced. Such actions promoted by secretive powerful officials including Harry Anslinger were also unlawfully hypocritical because scales of democratic justice are supposed to equate true and actual harm produced with true and actual punishment imposed. Trigger-happy shotgun-toting farmers motivated by Harry Anslinger and new government laws were committing much more violent and true demonstrable harms than merely transporting green herb marijuana plants. Where were the legal scales of democratic justice while such demonstrably harmful governments approved murders were occurring? The people being killed had not harmed anyone. The killers were motivated by government laws and related procedures. This is an example of how laws produce harms.

Similarly at this time, it was officially reported, "In considering all the marihuana cases in both General Sessions and Special Sessions courts, a total of 212 convictions, it is an impressive fact that only 30 offenders had been arrested before for drug charges. This does not argue very strongly for marihuana as a drug that initiates criminal careers."[504] While marihuana could not be truthfully related to producing demonstrable harms and promoting proven criminal careers, the same cannot be said for alcohol.

Alcohol is often involved with causing many true violent harms such as: murders, rapes, arsons, thefts and willful-damages. Truthful, official scientific research by Lloyd Shupe, for example shows direct significant relationships between people drinking alcohol and then doing actual demonstrable harms. "Shupe undertook a ten-year study in Columbus, Ohio, that involved a chemical analysis of the alcohol content of the trapped urine of all persons over 18 years of age arrested during or immediately following the alleged commission of a specific felony. Among the thirty persons arrested for murder, 67 percent had a blood alcohol concentration greater than .10.

A significant association with alcohol has also been found for aggravated assault. In an early study, Banay found assault to be the leading crime among inebriates incarcerated in Sing Sing prison between 1938 and 1940. . . .

Studies of forcible rape and other sex offences have also found a relationship between these violent crimes and alcohol. Lloyd Shupe, for example found that 45 percent of rape cases involved persons with a blood alcohol content of .10 or higher."[505] People drinking alcohol (God's worst enemy) caused many harms in North America. No similar truthful observations or substantiated conclusions were officially reported about people ingesting marihuana.

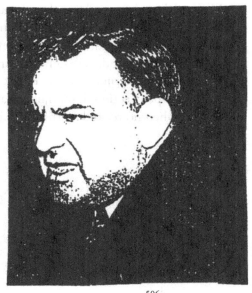

An important U.S. scientific and medical marihuana study, at this time was being objectively conducted by a committee of respected and knowledgeable individuals, at the request of New York's Mayor truth-seeking Mr. F.H. La Guardia. Mayor La Guardia preferred observing the truthful facts, rather than following biased advise of criminals who received reduced punishments and abstinances by merely blaming it on the 'weed'.

Footnote[506]

Some conclusions of this well organized, substantiated and scientifically conducted La Guardia Report are as follows:

"The practice of smoking marihuana does not lead to addiction in the medical sense of the word. . . .

The use of marihuana does not lead to morphine or heroin or cocaine addiction. . . .

Marihuana is not the determining factor in the commission of major crimes."[507] No truthful related harms were substantiated.

These objective and factual conclusions were from respected, educated and truth-seeking citizens. More relevant facts, truths, observations and conclusions have also been reported by this La Guardia Committee. Some additional testimony is as follows, "As the La Guardia Committee researchers found, marihuana quiets people and makes them more reflective. On the other hand, while alcohol may also quiet some people, it generally serves to weaken their inhibitions and may make them violent and unruly."[508]

Alcohol drinking also causes many family problems: poverty, arguments, overreactions, greed, revenge, rage, fights, jealousy, thefts and, "the dissolution of many marriages. . . . It is estimated that alcohol is the main factor in 75 percent of the domestic-relations actions brought into court. . . .

In sum, it is clear that alcohol is more harmful to both society and the individual than is marihuana. And yet, while alcohol is a legal means for people to seek relaxation . . . marihuana is not. This arbitrary classification is without rational basis and unfairly discriminates against marihuana devotees. They have been denied equal protection of the laws guaranteed by the Fourteenth Amendment to the U.S. Constitution."[509]

Man-made marijuana laws also violate Section Fifteen of the Canadian Charter of Rights and Freedoms. Sections 1 and 15 of the Charter guarantee each Canadian citizen the right to, "equal benefit of the law without discrimination."[510] Equal benefit of the law is violated when alcohol, a known multi-harm producer is given more favourable legal status than God's helpful and preferred marijuana plants. Marijuana laws are not demonstrably justified when compared to current alcohol laws. Also, as per Section 1 marijuana laws are not legally valid when they are not demonstrably justified, as when no related truthfully-substantiated proven harm is first produced.

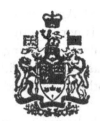

CANADIAN CHARTER OF RIGHTS AND FREEDOMS

Footnote[511]

When Pierre Elliott Trudeau signed the Canadian Charter of Rights and Freedoms in 1982, they became the highest level of laws in Canada's democratic constitution. The very first section of these important new laws describes that in Canada, laws are only valid if they can be demonstrably justified. The only way democratic government laws can be demonstrably justified is to address truthful harm. When no truthful, substantiated, measurable and proven harm is produced, it is beyond the legal limits allowed within the Canadian Charter of Rights and Freedoms for governments to interfere with peoples lives. Drinking alcohol produces more than 150 separate medical harms to peoples' bodies, including diseases, decays and deaths. Throughout history, documented records identify more than 150 separate medical benefits from ingesting natural marijuana plants, with no truthfully substantiated proven medical harms. Democratic governments are intended to be *for* the people. Encouraging a medically helpful product (150 times over) should have legal preference over encouraging a medically harmful product (150 times over). Logically, this amounts to 300 reasons why marijuana ingestion should be legally preferred to alcohol ingestion. The greatest good for the greatest number is another democratic principle denied, and this is not government *for* the people. Ingesting marijuana use has never produced even one truthfully substantiated case of lung cancer or death, whereas drinking alcohol has produced many cancers and deaths. Equal benefit of the law is not evident here. An unjust society exists with such basic discriminatory denials of fundamental justice.

Concerned members of the La Guardia Committee in 1942 concluded, "Marihuana does not of itself give rise to antisocial behavior. There is no evidence to suggest that the continued use of marihuana is a steppingstone to the use of opiates. Prolonged use of the drug does not lead to physical, mental or moral degeneration, nor have we observed any permanent deleterious effects from its continued use. Quite the contrary."[512] The previous three words are an important objective conclusion.

Similar understandings were also reported in India at this time. When describing effects of marijuana ingested by typical working people in India, scientific reports conclude that marijuana produces a sense of well-being, relieves fatigue and stimulates appetites.[513] Additional scientific analysis of marijuana showed similar results in North America. For example, "several studies carried out in the United States suggest that marihuana is not directly related to mental illness. Siler (1933) was unable to find cases of psychosis due to marihuana smoking, in a sample of several hundred American soldiers."[514] Whereas, no mental illness was produced with smoking marihuana, drinking alcohol produces delirium tremens among many other mental and physical diseases.

During World War Two, American kids were encouraged by the U.S. federal government to cultivate marihuana plants. Practical and knowledgeable officials realized that using marihuana plants would improve the chances of the Allies winning World War Two. By 1942,

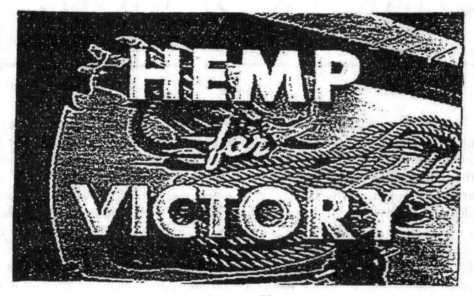

Footnote[515]

"marihuana, which had been outlawed in the United States . . . just four years earlier was suddenly safe enough for our government to ask the kids in the Kentucky 4-H club to grow the nation's 1943 seed supply. The youths were urged to grow at least half an acre, but preferably two acres of hemp each."[516]

During 1942-43, participating farmers were required, "to attend showings of the USDA film 'Hemp for Victory' sign that they had seen the film, and read a hemp cultivation booklet. Hemp harvesting machinery was made available at low or no cost. Five dollar tax stamps were available and 350,000 acres of cultivated hemp was the legal goal by 1943.

Farmers from 1942 through 1945 who agreed to grow hemp were waived from serving in the military, along with their sons."[517]

Freedman and Rockmore (1946) also failed to uncover any history of mental hospitalization in a sample of 300 soldiers, "who had been smoking marihuana for an average of seven years."[518] While many unusual unsubstantiated fictional fear stories against God's favoured marijuana plants were being sold in newspapers and other media at the time, not even one case of mental psychosis could be found in samples of several hundreds of American soldiers who regularly smoked marihuana.

In 1947, scientifically conducted experiments concluded that marihuana proved to be medically effective for successfully calming convulsions.[519] In 1949, marihuana, "was demonstrated to be effective in the control of seizures in several epileptic children who were unmanageable with the conventional drugs."[520] Helpful green herb marihuana provided successful medical uses for children, by relieving their harmful nervous disorders, that were 'unmanageable' with conventional pharmaceutical drugs. Once again, God's natural marihuana plants provided more medical effectiveness than man-made legal prescriptions. However, harmful laws still restrict and prohibit people from using medically helpful and effective marihuana goods, while legally allowing inferior, man-made substitutes to be used, some of which have produced demonstrably harmful side-effects to people. This does not demonstrate the greatest good *for* the greatest number of people. Equal benefit of the law is *not* evident here either.

It is arrogantly dangerous to prohibit divine directions, as God may well have severe long term punishments for those who devise or support man-made laws prohibiting the natural order, uses and goodness of God's resources and directions. What therefore God hath put together let no man put asunder.

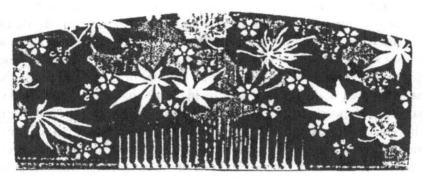

Footnote[521]

Additional scientific research at this time concludes, "no causal link has been demonstrated between the use of marihuana and the performance of other types of illegal behaviors."[522] Logical, rational, objective and analytical scientific studies conclude that ingestion of marihuana does not cause people to produce demonstrable harms. "The New York County Medical Society, and the President's Commission on Law Enforcement and the Administration of Justice have both found absolutely no evidence to indicate that marihuana causes criminal behaviour."[523] Informed and truthful testimony again shows that green herb marihuana does not cause demonstrable harms to be produced, contrary to some descriptions of untrue fiction stories and unsubstantiated excuses from proven harmful criminals.

Finally, even Harry Anslinger, "who was one of the prime movers to get marihuana banned noted before a congressional subcommittee in the 1950s, that marihuana was not a controlling factor in the commission of crimes."[524] Not only was marihuana not a controlling factor in the commission of true and violent crimes, but also scientific tests at this time conclude that marihuana use does not produce poor performance or loss of motivation. "In fact, numerous Army tests of the effects of cannabis on soldiers (through the 1950s and 60s) at Edgewood Arsenal, Maryland and elsewhere show no loss of motivation or performance after two years of heavy (military sponsored) smoking of marihuana. This study was repeated six more times by the military and dozens of times by universities, with the same or similar results. (Also, Panama/Siler study, Jamaican study, British Indian Hemp report.)"[525] Although many reasonable objective, truth-seeking officials agree that marihuana ingestion does not produce demonstrable harms, North American federal governments' laws still prohibit and criminalize marijuana's cultivation, transportation, sale, and general public beneficial uses. Marihuana remains legally publicly prohibited and condemned by federal governments' man-made laws, with no true substantiated and proven justifications. God can not be pleased with this practise, as he gave and directed people to use his natural green herb cannabis/marihuana plant goods, 'throughout the generations'.

Despite objective results of official scientific studies and reports concluding that marihuana use does not produce truthful harms, North American federal government lawmakers, without substantial demonstrable justification, surprisingly increased punishments against nonharmful people who cultivate, traffic, sell or ingest natural green herb marijuana. In the United States, the Federal Congress, at the behest of Harry Anslinger and his bureau, "passed the Boggs Act of 1951 and the Narcotic Control Act of 1956, which greatly increased the penalties for drug offences. By 1957 possession of marihuana carried a minimum sentence of two years for the first offence, five for the second, and ten for the third. First and second trafficking offences entailed minimum sentences of five and ten years respectively. With the exception of a first possession offense, all convictions carried a mandatory sentence with no chance of parole or probation."[526] Severe, true and harmful punishments that are *not* equated to the minor or no amount of actual and proven harm produced became criminally imposed against people for growing or nonharmfully using God's natural green herb marihuana plants. Hypocritical as it may be, these cruel and unusual punishments were quickly and secretively imposed in democratic countries proclaiming to be free, as in 'the "True North Strong and Free', 'Glorious and Free' and 'the Home of the Free'. Modern-age scales of democratic justice are harmfully imbalanced against God's helpful and preferred green herb marihuana plants, in terms of *not* equating punishments enforced to true and proven harms produced from marihuana users. When *no* related truthful harm is produced, laws are neither demonstrably justified nor constitutionally valid.

By 1949, Harry Anslinger and his associates started paying reward money to the public for identifying people who were using green herb marihuana plants, including: friends, neighbors, parents, grandparents and other family members. "The Bureau would use informants, some getting as much as $2,000 a crack to grease their tongues, and suddenly the Bureau's arm could reach into every . . . corner . . . of the country."[527] This cash payment method prompted many people to turn in their fellow citizens, *not* because they produced any true and measurable harm(s), but rather because of the substantial easy cash money available from the government. Why was this simple effective cash payment method not used against people harmfully drinking alcohol, as when alcohol was legally prohibited in the U.S. during the 1920s and early 30s?

As alluded to earlier, during the 1950s with no additional and demonstrable proven truths that green herb marihuana was producing actual damages to people or property, harmful legal punishments against nonharmful marihuana users were again arbitrarily intensified, without a public vote or referendum of approval. "For it was in fifties that the Draconian penalties associated with the drug laws were enacted amid an atmosphere of controlled hysteria."[528] Additional federal government hearings, "were held in 1951 by the House Ways and Means Committee, hearings that would eventually recommend legislation to shore up the criminal penalties for drug violations. A curious phenomenon developed at these hearings. The Bureau was forced after all these years to publicly acquiesce to the views of the respected members of the scientific community, with regard to marihuana. Dr. Harris Isbell, Director of Research at the Public Health Service Hospital in Lexington, Kentucky and a man who traditionally espoused the Bureau line admitted that many of the old myths were just that. Both in his paper to the House Committee and in his testimony before the Kefauver Committee, who held hearings to investigate organized crime that year, Isbell noted the relative innocuous quality to grass-smoking. He testified before the senators: Marihuana smokers generally . . . bother no one and have a good time. They do not stagger or fall. It has not been proved that smoking marihuana

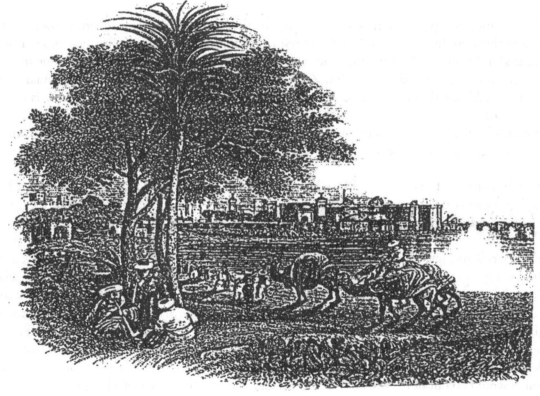

Footnote[529]

leads to crimes of violence, or to crimes of a sexual nature. Smoking marihuana has no unpleasant aftereffects and no dependence is developed on the drug."[530]

Unsubstantiated fearful fantacies about green herb marihuana were truthfully testified (at federal government hearings) to be officially described specifically as, mere myths, where a credible dictionary's definition of 'myth' is, "an invented story, something . . . having no existence in fact."[531] Irrespective of this truthful testimony, and without participative public support from a specific national democratic referendum or plebescite, severely imbalanced punishments are still being enforced against nonharmful pubic marihuana users. Conversely, no identical penalties (as in equal benefit of the law) are being actively applied against alcohol-drinking, a known producer of many true harms. Whereas, drinking alcohol has no similar severe legal man-made punishment schedule against it, the following official harmful punishment schedule was federally declared for convictions against the Marihuana Tax Act in 1951:

First Offense: Two to Five Years

Second Offense: Five to Ten Years

Third (and More): Ten to Twenty Years

Fine: Two Thousand Dollars[532]

Democratic scales of justice are supposed to equate the severity of the punishment to the severity of truthful harm(s) produced (from crimes). Consequently, it is demonstrably unjustified and harmfully imbalanced to impose a $2,000 punishment for a harmless action, when zero dollar value in actual harm is truthfully produced to a victim. Zero and two thousand are far from being equal, not to mention the additional oppresive punishment of two to twenty years in prison. First, it is cruel to withold or prevent someone from using beneficial medicine. Second, it is unusual to punish people for using traditionally helpful medicine. Cruel and unusual punishment is forbidden with Canada's Charter of Rights and Freedoms.

Fear propagator Harry Anslinger saved his job with the Marihuana Tax Act in 1951, but millions of people have since been unfairly punished, while many more millions have been denied legal access to numerous natural medical benefits from God's green herb marihuana plants.

Sly Harry Anslinger also secretively provided extra favours for influential people involved with making or approving related laws against God's marihuana plants. Cunning and controlling Harry Anslinger became very adept at quietly, "bestowing whatever favours he controlled on the gatekeepers, who could affect his tenure. Each time his appointment came up, Anslinger's elite army—the hanging judges . . . would surface from the woodwork beseeching the President and Secretary of the Treasurey. . . . Among his most vocal supporters were the pharmaceutical captains of industry, and the AMA, two of the groups that the Bureau in theory helped regulate. In return for their support, Anslinger would go out of his way to perform personal favours for his benefactors. For instance, one drug manufacturer wrote the Commissioner in 1952:

You mentioned your willingness to commend me to your departmental associates in a way that might expedite in some degree my baggage exam on returning from foreign countries."[533]

Actions of Harry Anslinger arbitrarily giving job-related favours to promote his personal career demonstrates 'influence peddling' and 'breach of trust'. Being that 'breach of trust' is a harmful (as in a fancy form of stealing) democratic crime, a valid legal action could have been applied against

Harry Anslinger each time he arranged an additional personal favour in return for extra support to advance his career? Breach of public trust is a serious, unethical and true democratic crime.

A respected and well-intentioned university professor, who had relevant official communications and experiences expresses similar descriptions of distrust and impropriety about Harry Anslinger. Professor Alfred Lindesmith from Indiana University advises, "You can't believe what Anslinger says" . . . Lindesmith cautions. "An entrepreneur and a politician like Anslinger is playing a game, and it was perfectly obvious to me when I met him at the White House Conference."[534] Harry Anslinger became an untrusted unethical opportunist playing games with peoples' lives.

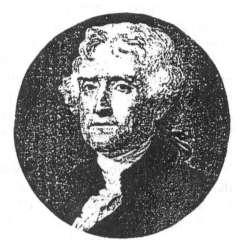

Footnote[535]

Modern medicine may have evolved into an actual harm producer, legally encouraging pharmaceuticals with harmful side-effects, while also legally preventing public access to a traditionally helpful medical resource (marihuana) with no harmful side-effects. Two other U.S. fathers of democracy, 'for' the people, Dr. Benjamen Rush (George Washington's personal physician and signer of the Declaration of Independence) and President Thomas Jefferson both foresaw intentional legal misuse of ongoing public access to helpful and nonharmful medicines. Dr. Rush humanely warned that unless medical freedom is constitutionally guaranteed, medicine will eventually become 'an undercover dictatorship' in which the art of healing will be restricted to one class of men while equal privileges are denied to others.[536]

Democratic principles of fundamental justice require *equal* benefit of the law, *not* playing games with peoples lives.

Anslinger's aggressive attention about criminalizing marihuana users with man-made laws and horrendously excessive punishments, also diverted attention away from drinking alcohol, a true and proven multi-harm producer. Harry Anslinger's department recommended and enforced extremely severe punishments against marihuana participants, using the unsubstantiated, untrue and incorrect man-made legal classification that marihuana was a narcotic, when truthfully it is not a narcotic in any medical sense, nor was it ever proven to be a true narcotic in any official previous context.

That marihuana is incorrectly legally classified as a narcotic is substantiated by Doctor Rod M. Mikuriya of San Francisco, who explains that marihuana, "is not a narcotic in the medical sense. Since it is not physiologically addicting, says Dr. Mikuriya there are no withdrawal pains. There is little or no buildup or tolerance that would lead to the use of increasing doses, as is the case with true narcotics (opium and its refined extracts, heroin, morphine, codeine) and their synthetic substitutes."[537] But despite medical truths, unfair laws continue with unjust punishments against nonharmful public participants who beneficially use God's helpful green herb marihuana plants.

Even the U.S. Whitehouse Conference on Narcotics and Other Drug Abuse in 1962 recognized the unjust penalties imposed against users, growers and sellers of medically beneficial marijuana. "It is the opinion of the panel that the hazards of marihuana per se have been exaggerated and the long criminal sentences imposed on occasional users or possessors are in poor social perspective."[538] Other federal officials in the U.S. expressed similar more just and true legal actions about marihuana. "Noting the relatively minor nature of a marihuana offense, the President's Advisory Commission in 1963 suggested the elimination of all mandatory sentences relating to it."[539] It was also officially stated, "Crimes which could be shown to the satisfaction of a court of law to be linked with the use of marihuana ought to be dealt with about the way that crimes arising from the use of alcohol are handled."[540] This would have at least reduced the significant legal discrimination factor between marihuana and alcohol users. Such rational recommendations, however were disregarded, as helpful green herb marihuana is still criminalized and harmfully punished against by democratic governments.

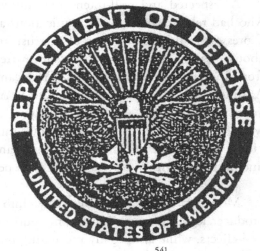

Footnote[541]

The U.S. Department of Defense also truthfully reported on medical uses of marihuana during the 1960s. Positive results were observed with: lowering high blood pressure, reducing pain, decreasing anxiety, and reducing depression.[542]

Other areas of the world at this time similarily received valuable medical results from using green herb marihuana plants. Well-intentioned and constructive-minded eastern areas of the world, 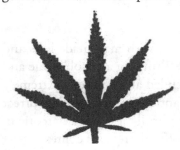 for example reported successful results when using marihuana for relieving medical harms including: headaches, nervous tension and malaria. With some medical uses of marihuana, "cooked leaves which have been dried in the sun are used in quantities of several grams per bowl of water. This . . . helps especially to combat migraines and stiffness, taken before sleep and before meals it relaxes the nerves. . . . This beneficial medical action is recognized . . . by the official pharmacopoeia of these countries."[543]

To cure malaria, it is recorded that affected individuals inhale one kilogram of male and female plants, "twice a day until the end of the crisis. The same amount of hemp and water in a preparation taken in 2cc. doses before each meal sometimes replaces the inhalation method but is not as effective."[544] Medical records also disclose that sandalwood and marihuana plants, "have a beneficial effect on the functioning of the heart, the liver and the lungs, this is taken in the form of tea."[545] It is unjust imposing punishments on people who nonharmfully use green herb marijuana plants to improve their medical harms. Such legalized public prevention of helpful medicine is an unjustified crime against humanity.

Doctor Edward Bloomquist (University of Southern California) recognizes this unjust disparity on the scales of democratic justice, that are supposed to equate the punishment to the true and actual value of the harm(s) produced. He logically explains, "The problem is that in our zeal we have in some areas permitted and promoted laws that are disproportionately severe to the crime involved."[546] When no true and actual harm is done, no true and actual punishment is justified. Such democratic justice is reasonable, easy to understand and fair.

Other U.S. federal government officials also began recognizing considerable differences between the severe punishments being imposed, as compared to the related proven and actual harm(s) produced. "Both the Ad Hoc Panel on Drug Abuse in 1962 and the Advisory Commission on Narcotic and Drug Abuse in 1963 tersely questioned the existing penalties."[547] Official U.S. federal government statements describe significant differences between marihuana and *true* narcotics such as morphine and alcohol. Official records of President Kennedy's Advisory Commission on Narcotic and Drug Abuse conclude, "The present federal narcotics and marihuana laws equate the two drugs. Any offender whose crime is sale of a marihuana reefer is subject to the same term of imprisonment as the peddler selling heroin. . . . For one thing . . . marihuana . . . does not create physical dependency."[548] Theodore Barber of a Massachusetts State hospital confirms this medical conclusion, "Marihuana and other forms of cannabis do not produce addiction as defined by tolerance, physical dependence and a withdrawal syndrome (Chopra & Chopra, 1957). There is no evidence that users become physiologically tolerant to the effects of cannabis so that they have to increase the dose in order to obtain the desired effects. There is no evidence that cannabis produces a change in the user's physiological processes so that he requires continued administration of the drug in order to function properly."[549] Marihuana does not produce addiction, tolerance, withdrawal pains, nausea, headaches or constipation, as do *true* and harmful narcotics including: morphine, alcohol, heroin, codiene and cocaine.

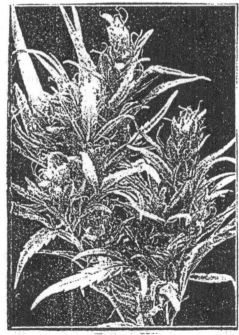

Footnote[551]

A comprehensive U.S. government report published in 1944, the LaGuardia Report also truthfully observes and concludes that marihuana use does not lead to addiction of *true* narcotics, such as opium and morphine. This scientifically conducted truth seeking study was prepared by respected and relevant committee members, with assistance from the New York City Police Department. After much careful scientific observations and objective analysis, this official report concludes, "The use of marihuana does not lead to morphine, or heroin or cocaine addiction."[550] Because, natural green herb marihuana is *not* a narcotic, and does *not* lead to true narcotic addiction, it should not mistakenly be legally classified as a narcotic, since such behaviour is inconsistent with truthful reality, reasonable logic, democratic liberty, and fundamental justice.

Additional conclusions of this government prepared LaGuardia Report disclose that marihuana, "is not the determining factor in the commission of major crimes. . . .

The publicity concerning the catastrophic effects of marihuana smoking in New York City is unfounded."[552] Untrue, horrible fear stories were published against God's helpful green herb marihuana plants.

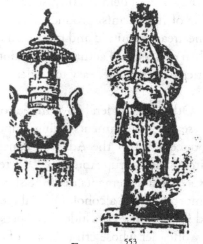

In other areas of the world, favourable observations and conclusions continued being recorded concerning people ingesting marihuana. In the mid 1950s, two respected international research scientists Chopra and Chopra reported results of an extensive cannabis survey in India, trying to find a relationship between people physically ingesting marihuana and then producing truthful demonstrable harm(s) such as actually damaging people or property. Their extensive objective results conclude that human consumption of marihuana actually reduces crimes as they report, "The result of continued and excessive use of these drugs in our experience in India is to make the individual timid, rather than to lead him to commit violent crimes."[554]

Footnote [553]

Similar substantiated conclusions were reported in England during the 1960s. This, "British Government (1968) study could find no evidence that the increase in the consumption of cannabis in Britain is causing aggressive antisocial behaviour or crimes. It also appears that the crime rate has not increased in areas of the United States where marihuana use has increased tremendously in recent years (Simmons, 1967)."[555] During the 1960s, "legions of American researchers had positive indications with using cannabis for: asthma, glaucoma, nausea from chemotherapy, anorexia, tumors and epilepsy, as well as a general use antibiotic. Cumulative results showed evidence or favourable anomalies occurring for: Parkinson's disease, anorexia, multiple sclerosis and muscular dystrophy."[556]

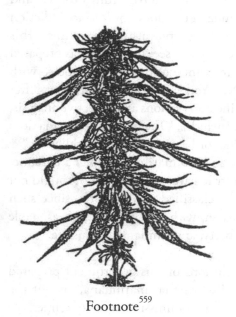

Footnote [559]

Multiple Sclerosis (MS) is a medical disorder in which nerves throughout a person's body, "are attacked by a person's own immune system. MS is a chronic illness which can get worse over time. Many people with MS have reported good results from smoking marihuana at the onset of an attack. Because marihuana goes into the body's system quickly when smoked, it is the preferred method of ingestion."[557] Another medical report concludes, "smoking cannabis has proven to be a major source of relief for multiple sclerosis which affects the nervous system, and is characterized by muscular weakness, tremors, etc."[558] As green herb marihuana has been shown to improve medical disorders while not producing demonstrable harms, freedom of choice to healthfully participate is not legally available.

In the United States some official recommendations were being made regarding removal of man-made laws and

108

punishments against green herb marihuana participants. For example, the 1967 President's Crime Commission, "made some strong recommendations for revising marihuana laws. . . . Task Force member Dr. M. Rosenthal proposed that criminal sanction against use and possession be entirely removed."[560]

During the 1960s, other public groups of well-intentioned people in the United States also expressed support for eliminating laws against marihuana. The National Review, "a journal of extreme-right conservative opinion published an article asking, "Should We Legalize Pot?" that was answered with a resounding, "Yes!"[561] This demonstrates electoral support for legalizing nonharmful marihuana uses.

Another reasonable U.S. publication, the New Republic, "has long called for the repeal of marihuana laws."[562] As well, in Washington D.C., "the President's Commission on Crime strongly urged that present penalties on marihuana be eased."[563] This is primarily because no causal relationship could be scientifically proven to exist between ingesting marihuana and truthfully producing demonstrable harm(s) to people or property.

In vivid contrast, personal consumption of alcohol has often been related to producing demonstrable harms including true public crimes with measurable and identifiable damages. During the 1960s in the U.S., "the President's Commission on Law Enforcement and the Administration of Justice, and the British Advisory Committee on Drug Dependence noted the circumstantial evidence link between marihuana and crime is much weaker than the known link between alcohol and crime."[564] The known link between alcohol and crime with its true demonstrable harms has been identified at least thousands of times in North America especially since 1933.

People from other countries in the world during the 1960s continued reporting nonharmful results with using green herb marihuana. "Similarly, studies in Brazil and Nigeria have failed to find a causal relationship between cannabis and criminal activities."[565] When no true and demonstrable harm(s) are produced from smoking or otherwise physically ingesting marihuana plant goods, no related harmful punishment is legally valid to impose. Demonstrable justification and truthfully proven harm are required first.

However, when actual harm is done, or harm-maker(s) claim that marihuana consumption caused their harmful actions, such harm-making criminal(s) should be legally prohibited from using marijuana. But only these harm-making people should be prohibited and punished for their harmful actions. All other nonharmful users within the democracy should not be punished or restricted. Punishments are only legally applicable to harm-makers, not anyone else. When no proven demonstrable harm is truthfully produced no related punishment is lawful to impose.

Whereas, marihuana plants are not medically, scientifically or truthfully related to producing actual demonstrable harms, the same cannot be said for legalized alcohol drinks. In an official U.S. Court of Law near the beginning of the 1970s, presenting truths and evidence, reliable testimony clearly concludes, "alcohol incapacitates millions—there are some five million alcoholics in this country, and as I have noted earlier 20 percent of the patients admitted to state mental hospitals were admitted because of alcoholic problems, marihuana on the other hand is harmless."[566] Harmless is how an objective observant official describes marihuana in an American Court of Law, whose primary function is obtaining and providing the truth, the whole truth, and nothing but the truth, so help us God.

Federal government authorities from various western world countries confirm that public marijuana consumption by itself (not mixed with ingesting alcohol or other contaminants) does *not* produce demonstrable harms. In the United Kingdom for example, the Wooton Commission (1968) concludes, "The taking of cannabis had not so far been regarded, even by the severest critics, as a direct cause of serious crime. The Le Dain Commission in Canada came to similar conclusions."[567]

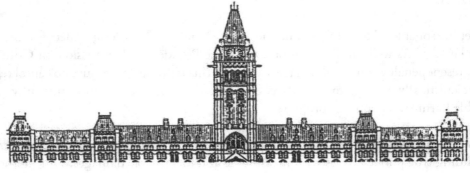

Footnote[568]

The Canadian federal government, "appointed a commission of enquiry into the nonmedical use of drugs in May 1969. It became popularly called the Le Dain Commission, after its chairman Gerald Le Dain, Dean of Osgoode Hall Law School in Toronto. In its 320 page Interim Report which appeared in April 1970, the Commission described the need to legalize the simple possession of cannabis . . . in terms of the cost of prohibition. Enforcement of drug laws the Commission said, costs far too much in individual and social terms including destruction of young lives and growing disrespect for the law. . . . The Commission is of the opinion that no one should be liable to imprisonment for simple possession. . . . The illicit status of cannabis invites exploitation by criminal elements and other abuses. . . . It is said cannabis should be made available under government controlled conditions of quality and availability."[569] More truthful and scientific research attributes, "applied to marijuana smokers by the Le Dain Commission and others are: talkative, cheerful, relaxed and disinhibited, cool and composed attitude, peaceful, feelings of creativity, (clears the brain for thought) thoughts more intuitive, and empathy for others."[570]

As conclusions of officially, scientifically and medically substantiated reports describe the harmless and helpful natures of marijuana, especially in relation to alcohol, democratic laws *for* the people, *for* the person, *for* life, *for* liberty, *for* security, and *for* happiness are not actively evident or demonstrated here.

From injustice and medical perspectives, marijuana suddenly became secretively and incorrectly legally classified as a harmful narcotic, during the 1920s and 30s in Canada and the United States. In neither of these democratic countries was a specific public majority-vote ever officially conducted to approve this legal change in man-made definition. After thousands of consecutive years with beneficial public uses, secretively contrived, misguided man-made laws suddenly and unjustifiably classified God's helpful and natural green herb marijuana as an illegal harmful 'narcotic' when in truthful fact it is harmless.

Near the beginning of the 1960s in the United States, "Dr. Stanley Yolles, while serving as Director of the National Institute of Mental Health pointed out some striking contrasts between fact and fable. He prepared a chart listing these distinctions.

FABLE: Marihuana is a narcotic.

FACT: Marihuana is not a narcotic except by statute. Narcoties are opium or its derivatives—like heroin and morphine and some synthetic chemicals with opium-like activity."[571]

True narcotics are known to produce demonstrable physical harms to various bodily organs, whereas marihuana does not do this. More official U.S. court testimony concludes, "Marihuana does not produce a physical dependence requiring constant use to prevent painful withdrawal symptoms. It also does not produce tolerance, that is more of the drug is not needed each time to produce the desired results."[572] These are credible and significant true differences, logically and demonstrably separating marihuana as *not* being a true and harmful narcotic such as: morphine, alcohol, opium, heroin, cocaine, codeine and chloral-hydrate.

Additional official U.S. court testimony about 1970 explains, "No Your Honor. Unlike alcohol which is physically dangerous and can lead to death, marihuana is not dangerous. An associate medical examiner in New York City reports that in his extensive autopsy experience with hundreds of marihuana users, he was unable to find any evidence of physical deterioration caused by marihuana. Furthermore he reported, and the President's Commission on Law Enforcement and the Administration of Justice found as well, that no deaths have been attributable to marijuana use. Both the La Guardia Committee Report and the extensive study conducted in the 1890s, by the Indian Hemp Drug

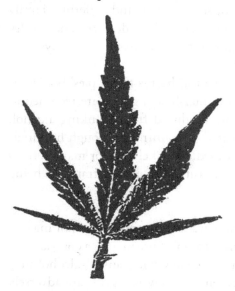

Commission indicate that the long-term consumption of moderate doses of marihuana is not harmful."[573] The Indian Hemp Drug Commission Report of 1893-1894 consisting of, "nine volumes and 3,698 pages is by far the most complete and systematic study undertaken to date."[574] All credible, objective, scientific and substantiated studies show marihuana uses to be helpful and harmless. Harry Anslinger and other secretive powerful officials prevented public medical uses of God's preferred green herb marijuana plants. "Vengeance is mine sayeth the Lord" and people supporting laws against marijuana have this to face some day, perhaps not too far away.

Additional court testimony concludes, "a 1946 study of 310 men in the Army, who had used marihuana on the average for seven years revealed no mental or physical deterioration."[575] Small samples can reliably predict behaviours of large populations. With no deterioration occurring in a small sample size of 310 men, large populations are statistically reported to be very similar. George

Washington, a well-respected soldier and President of the population of the United States received an attractive vote of 69-0 from his Electoral College political peers, before becoming the first president of the United States.[576] A score of 310-0 is even more impressive.

1961, the upsidedown year witnessed a severe setback to nonharmful users of God's preferred medically helpful green herb marijuana plants, significantly imbalancing the scales of fundamental justice. "In 1961, at a time when the drug was still barely in use in Canada, the Narcotic Control Act made simple possession of marijuana punishable by up to seven years in prison. By the end of that decade . . . more than 10,000 Canadians a year were being arrested for possession."[577]

Also in 1961, without specific approval from the majority of Canadian voters, Canada signed the U.N. convention on Narcotic Drugs and unjustifiably increased punishments for, "cultivating and importing marijuana."[578] 1961 was a bad year for public liberty around the world. During this infamous year the Berlin Wall also went up, but at least it came down in 1989.

Even current harmful punishments for cultivating or trafficking are irrationally imbalanced on traditional scales of fundamental justice. A reporter from Nova Scotia in 2002 demonstrably explains, "Last week I wrote here about a young offender who was sentenced to two years in youth jail for brutally murdering another teen with a baseball bat. Also last week Michael Patriquen of Sackville was sentenced to six years hard time for marijuana trafficking and possession. There's something very wrong with this picture."[579]

Deaths on highways often result from people drinking alcohol. More than 25,000 North Americans were killed in motor vehicle accidents attributed to alcohol-drinking in 1971.

Similarly, an official study identifying harmful costs from drinking alcohol, "generated a first approximation of the economic cost of alcohol abuse in 1971 of some $25 billion. . . . But, a dollar figure cannot convey the very real nontangible losses sustained, such as pain and suffering, family anguish and other adverse consequences that affect the family and friends of the deceased and society in general."[580] Drinking alcohol demonstrably harms people and property in many tragic ways.

While alcohol-drinking continues causing many truthful medical harms to peoples' bodies, at the opposite or healthy end of the human nutritional spectrum, marihuana goods are recorded as being effective for improving dangerous medical harms, many produced from drinking alcohol. Related, "U.S. government research (1966 to 1976) had indicated or confirmed through hundreds of studies that 'natural' crude cannabis was the best and safest medicine of choice for many serious health problems."[581] Again, God's helpful marihuana plants are truthfully demonstrated as being safe, effective and harmless.

People drinking alcohol also tend to become involved with fire and arson(s). "Alcohol may be related to fire and its consequences in two ways. On the one hand, alcohol abuse may be a contributing cause of fire in the first place. On the other hand, given a fire—whatever its cause—alcohol may well serve to intensify its adverse consequences because judgement and physical skills are adversely affected even at low levels of blood alcohol content. . . . W. Slater Hollis studied twenty-nine fire deaths of persons aged 16 to 20, that occurred over a period of eight years in Memphis Tennessee.

Hollis found the relationship between blood alcohol content and the number of fire deaths to be quite significant. . . . In fact he concluded that the primary cause of these fire deaths was alcohol consumption. Hollis compared the autopsy results with fire, police and medical examiner's reports and noted, "alcohol ingestion is the normal accompaniment of fire deaths and the most common attributed primary cause of death."[582] Drinking alcohol not only destroys people internally with demonstrable harms, but in many cases alcohol and fire kill people externally with searing and vicious flames that painfully hurt, sizzle, mutilate and destroy. Fire and heat from spontaneous human combustion have also killed people who had previously ingested alcohol. Vapours burn.

On the healthy side of the life-death spectrum, marihuana consumption was not mentioned as relating to even one death. This is because natural marijuana has been truthfully known for improving and helping peoples' bodily functions and processes. "One of the more frequently stated reasons for continuing to use cannabis moderately is the sense of well-being, relaxation and relief from tension experienced. . . . (Chopra & Chopra, 1957, Indian Hemp Drug Commission, 1894). Another factual reason for its continued use is relief from boredom, frustration and depression (McGlothlin et al., 1970)."[583]

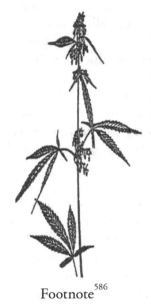

Footnote[586]

"The meteoric rise in the number of young citizens with criminal records began to force a rethink of marijuana laws."[584] A report by the Canadian federal Le Dain Commission in 1972 concluded that criminal prohibition of marijuana was a misguided case of injustice, and recommended more fair and reasonable laws be designed and approved by parliament. When discussing behaviours of people consuming marijuana, as in smoking it for example, the Canadian Le Dain Committee concludes, "the positive values people find in . . . the experience bear a striking similarity to traditional religious values including concern with the soul or inner self. The spirit of renunciation, the emphasis on openness, and the closely-knit community are part of it but this is definately a sense of identification with something larger, something to which one belongs as part of the human race."[585] Indeed, consuming marijuana tends to make a person more humane, compassionate, listen better, and be concerned with adding value without doing harm(s) to people or property.

More helpful medical uses of marijuana have also been identified. One valuable application has been with cancer patients. Beneficial effects of marijuana demonstrated over a short period of time were: "stimulation of appetite, euphoria, increased sense of well-being, mild analgesia, and an indifference to pain which reduced the need for opiates."[587] Dr. Thomas Ungerleider, head of California's Marihuana For Cancer Research Program (1979 to 1984) similarly concludes, results from related scientific studies show, "Marihuana is the best agent for control of nausea in cancer chemotherapy."[588]

Other medical reports likewise conclude, "Marijuana is used to stimulate appetite during chemo and radiation therapy for cancer patients. Marijuana stimulates appetite both when eaten and when smoked, although the medicinal effects last longer when the grass is eaten. Patients suffering from nausea may smoke a joint initially, then follow up by eating marijuana when they can hold food down.

Marijuana is also helpful for pain relief associated with cancer. Eating marijuana is more effective and long lasting for relieving pain providing relief for up to 12 hours. Marijuana has been adopted by cancer patients, because it is more effective with fewer side effects than many of the pharmaceutical drugs available. . . . The nausea from chemotherapy can be life threatening in itself, as many patients experience rapid declines in weight from an inability to keep food down."[589] Marijuana is a unique, reliable, medically improving plant even for sorrowful cancerous patients.

More studies, "by Joanna Budwig, M.D. (nominated for Nobel Peace Prize every year since 1979) have shown unparalleled results in the use of essential fatty acids for the treatment of terminal cancer patients. What are essential fatty acids? The term 'essential' is the tip-off. Truly, there can be no life anywhere without the essential oils: linoleic and linolenic acids. These essential oils support the immune system and guard against viral and other insults to the immune system. . . . What is the richest source of the essential oil? . . . the seeds of the cannabis hemp plant. The seeds contain 25% LNA acid and 51% LA acid. What better proof of the life-giving values of the . . . seed."[590] God directed that people eat herb seeds as meat.

Additional support for using marijuana in helpful treatments with cancer patients came during the 1980s, from an official U.S. judge. A Drug Enforcement Administration judge, calling marihuana, "one of the safest therapeutically active substances known to man" recommended yesterday that the drug be made legally available for some medical purposes including treatment of cancer patients.

If adopted, the opinion by Judge Francis L. Young could soon allow doctors to lawfully prescribe marihuana.[591] Improving cancerous conditions is a crucial curative characteristic of marihuana, as an obvious scarcity of successful medicines exist for effectively eliminating cancer. Appropriate applications of green herb marijuana could indeed prove to be a reliable cure for cancer, given truthful, unrestricted and unharmful efforts to freely study and confirm this objective.

Another reputable medical report has more favourable news about marijuana plants. "Extracts of unripe cannabis have also been demonstrated to have antibiotic activity against certain bacteria and fungi. . . . Other THC analogues may prove to be valuable agents for the treatment of high blood pressure and uncontrollable fevers."[592] These same helpful results are *not* similarly observed from drinking alcohol. Yet, harm-producing alcohol is legally available, while God's multi-beneficial marijuana is not. This true discrimination produces a significant imbalance on the scales of fundamental justice.

Additional official international health reports describe more successful medical uses of marijuana. In Czechoslovakia for example, research studies for more than twenty consecutive years, comparing hundreds of different plants, resulted in selection of marijuana, "as the most promising antibiotic out of hundreds of species, and it is now used for a whole range of diseases. Dr. Miller mentioned ongoing work in raising seizure thresholds in epileptics and lowering intraocular pressure in glaucoma.

In Canada, there are reports of people taking cannabis to reduce secondary symptoms of flu or colds."[593] In the United States, a similar medical report concludes that marihuana plant components are, "useful in the treatment of glaucoma patients, because marihuana reduces intraocular pressure."[594]

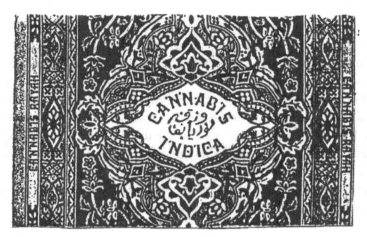

Footnote[595]

Marijuana smoked, or applied as a herbal pack or poultice is also the best muscle relaxant, back spasm medicine and antispasmodic medication."[596] An objective medical report concludes, "marijuana is helpful in calming many kinds of spasms, such as those related to spinal cord injuries and muscle spasms. Smoking, rather than eating is preferred because relief comes quickly when taken in this manner. Eating marijuana is more effective for pain relief."[597]

Ingesting marijuana is also a successful medical treatment for ulcers. "Stomach acid output decreases after the consumption of cannabis, which recommends it for the treatment of peptic ulcers, colitis, ileitis, spastic colon and gastritis. Preparations of cannabis were used for these purposes in the 1890s."[598]

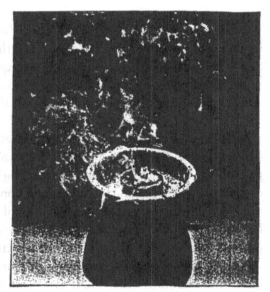

Other medical records confirm marijuana's beneficial use for treating epilepsy. One of the traditional, "uses of cannabis preparations was as an anticonvulsant to control seizures of all kinds. Epilepsy is a chronic disease, that when active is characterized by large or small seizures. There is a strong movement of people with this illness, who are medicating themselves with marijuana. This is because marijuana, in many situations seems more effective than the medicines available, with fewer side effects. Strong barbiturates and anticonvulsant drugs like Dilantin are frequently prescribed for epilepsy.

Footnote[599]

Though smoking marijuana can be used to quickly get the drug into the body when needed, eating marijuana is helpful for long term relief."[600]

Smoking marijuana is also healthy for human lungs. "Cannabis is the best natural expectorant to clear the human lungs of smog, dust and . . . phlegm. Marihuana smoke effectively dilates the airways of the lungs, the bronchi opening them to allow more oxygen into the lungs."[601] Natural marijuana smoke attracts phlegm for expectoration to rid the body of biologically electron poor substances.

In the eastern world, marijuana is reported to be a successful medication that, "cures hemorrhoids and polyps of the throat, intestines and the sex organs. . . . Cannabis is frequently used to stimulate the appetite of sick people and make them sleep. In cigarettes mixed with tobacco, it relieves asthma. Its use to counteract diarrhea and dysentery is equally common."[602] Beneficial marijuana preparations also facilitate contractions during difficult periods of childbirth.[603] Kernels of marijuana seeds have been effectively used in medical preparations, "to combat loss of memory and mental confusion, aging, ailments due to 'unhealthy breezes' that engender psoriasis with dark spots, decongest the organism, eliminate blood wastes, cure dysmenorrhoea, and produce a feeling of well-being after childbirth. In obstetrics, if the presentation of the child is awkward, twenty-one kernels boiled in water have the power of replacing him in the normal position."[604]

Green herb marijuana plants have additionally been used, "to cure stomach ailments . . . the swollen stomach (of cattle as well as people) the sick person drinks a preparation from the male and female leaves."[605] Several impressive medical uses of marijuana are internationally recorded.

God's green herb marijuana also has a reliable reputation for reducing tumors. A tumor is a mass of swollen tissue in a body. Researchers at the Medical College of Virginia have concluded, "Cannabis is an incredibly successful herb for reducing many types of tumors both benign and malignant (cancerous)."[606]

Tried, true and trusted medical uses of marijuana plants suddenly became prohibited with man-made laws and severe punishments in North America, at almost the same time as when the United States and many other countries began experiencing violent harms of World War Two. With no public approval from a specific democratic national marihuana referendum and at the behest of Harry Anslinger, "and his crowd, marihuana was dropped from the Pharmacopoeia in 1941."[607]

The Marihuana Tax Act began its official public imposition on September 1, 1937. Within a short time and some harmful man made decisions with secretively contrived legislation, God's preferred green herb marihuana suddenly became legally publicly prohibited from medically helping people. Compared to the previous ten thousand consecutive years of world history, this sudden legal denial of helpful medicine was cruel and unusual treatment. Secretively depriving the public of natural beneficial medicine is *not* democracy *for* the people. From a humane perspective alone, not allowing people to use a helpful and curative medicine is also uncaring, unethical, callous, selfish, morally demented and malicious. Legally prohibiting people from beneficially using curative and comforting medicine is not only cruel and unusual man made behaviour, but as previously mentioned it is also inhumane and immoral because these man made laws intentionally deny corrective medical goods to people who are trying to improve their lives in a free country. In Canada, everyone is constitutionally guaranteed democratic rights and freedoms advocating life, liberty, security and joy. Also, such unjust and unnatural laws against nonharmful public users of marijuana are contrary to God's directions, and we must all reconcile with God in the not too distant future. Among other important reasons, it's much safer to be supportive of God's intentions long before judgement day arrives. God also condemns crimes against humanity such as witholding naturally helpful medicine from the public.

Although North American marijuana prohibition laws have been somewhat modified since the 1960s, marijuana plants are still not readily and legally available to the general public as healthy uses

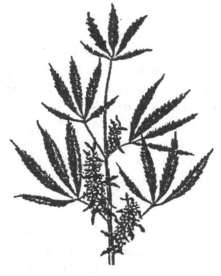

for medicines, foods and clothing. An amendment to the Canadian Narcotic Control Act in 1969 declared possession of marijuana to remain a criminal offence, but now to be classified as a 'summary conviction' criminal offence. For a marijuana possession conviction there developed a different punishment method of a monetary fine, as an option to imprisonment or a suspended sentence.

In 1972, The Criminal Code in Canada was changed to include conditional and absolute discharges as options for punishments including imprisonments.[608]

Although some legal modifications have occurred in Canada, unjust man-made marijuana laws with harmful punishments remain described and enforced as being criminal activities with criminal punishments and criminal records. This is not consistent with God's directions of, "Behold, I have given you every herb . . . which is upon the face of all the earth . . . to

Footnote[609]

you it shall be for meat. . . . I have given every green herb for meat. . . . and thou shalt eat the herb of the field."[610] North American federal governments' laws traditionally value and advocate life, liberty, security, happiness and trust in God.

At a U.S. federal court in 1970, a humane and knowledgeable medical authority, Mr. Smith testified before Mr. Justice Spencer as follows:

"First of all, marihuana does not harm the individual user. . . .

The Chief Justice: Is marihuana physically harmful?

Mr. Smith: No, Your Honor. Unlike alcohol which is physically dangerous . . . marihuana is not dangerous. . . . There is no evidence that the use of marihuana causes criminality. This has been borne out by everybody who has studied the situation. . . . Scientific studies have consistently indicated that marihuana does not seriously adversely affect the user either in the short term or in the long term."[611]

In 1972, an official Canadian federal government report reconfirmed that marijuana is *not* a true narcotic. Results of the Le Dain Report conclude, "It was established that cannabis was not a 'narcotic' in any pharmacological or behavioural sense. . . . Its use did not cause people to become criminals or moral degenerates. (Le Dain, 1972; Shafer, 1972)."[612] Even though, marijuana has been medically, behaviorally, morally, scientifically, historically and pharmacologically established *not* to be a true narcotic, helpful green herb marijuana remains wrongfully included in the Canadian Narcotic Control Act, with criminal records and significantly disproportionate unjust punishments preventing nonharmful people from obtaining trustworthy jobs, for example. Marijuana is not a true and harmful narcotic. Consequently, it is incorrect, unjustified and undemocratic to continue harming people with wrongful punishments from the Canadian Narcotic Control Act.

A similar scenario exists in the United States, where it has been truthfully concluded that marihuana does not cause a medical threat to public health. It is officially reported, "the National Commission on Marihuana and Drug Abuse reached the following conclusion in its 1972 report. From what is now known about the effects of marihuana, its use at the present level does not constitute a major threat to public health. . . . We believe that experimental or intermittent use of this drug carries minimal risk to public health and should not be given overzealous attention."[613] Because it should not be given overzealous attention, natural green herb marihuana should *not* be legally classified as a criminal narcotic when: medically, scientifically, morally, behaviourally, factually, historically and pharmacologically it has been determined *not* to be a narcotic. Similarly, marihuana has also been officially shown *not* to have any of the demonstrably harmful characteristics of true and harmful narcotics such as heroin, alcohol and morphine.

During 1972, an encouraging federal report in the United States recommended that possession of marihuana be decriminalized. Nothing, however was constructively mentioned about decriminalizing cultivation, trafficking or general nonharmful public consumption of marihuana as God intended.

The National Commission on Marihuana and Drug Abuse, "recommended that possession of marihuana for personal use and nonprofit distribution should be decriminalized. . . . The commission's proposal was endorsed by a long list of newspapers and by numerous organizations including the: American Bar Association, American Medical Association, American Public Health Association, National Education Association, Consumers Union, National Council of Churches, National Conference of Commissioners on Uniform State Laws, and American Academy of Pediatrics."[614] Many prudent and reliable people have expressed solid support and official recommendations for publicly using green herb marihuana.

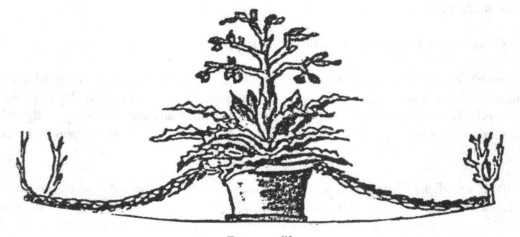

Footnote[615]

However, unjust criminal laws and harmful punishments remain in place against cultivating, purchasing, selling, marketing, transporting, trafficking, importing, exporting, and/or publicly ingesting marihuana in North America. A rare but noticeable improvement in the direction of removing man-made laws against marihuana plant users occurred in 1972, when many U.S. states, "reduced possession of marihuana from a felony to a misdemeanor."[616] However, this applied only to possession of marihuana which is still an unlawful crime, only its man-made legal classification changed from felony to misdemeanor. Additional unjust criminal laws and punishments are still in place in North America and many other areas of the world for: cultivating, trafficking, selling, marketing, importing, exporting and/or ingesting marijuana plants. Again, this is immensely inconsistent with initial instructions from God. "Behold, I have given you every herb. . . . to you it shall be for meat. . . . I have given every green herb for meat. . . . and thou shalt eat the herb of the field."[617] History has told us many times that God has much punishable abilities against those who thwart his instructions.

When no truthful and demonstrable harm has been produced, no harmful punishment should legally be imposed. In the 1970s, this basic moral principle was supported by more official U.S. court testimony. "We seek reaffirmation of what the late Mr. Justice Brandeis has characterized as "the most comprehensive of rights, and the right most valued by civilized man—the right to be let alone."[618] It was humanely explained that the real role of government should not be to tell us, "what we can read, think, eat, drink or even smoke—without demonstrating that the clear and present danger of our actions so imperils society or endangers ourselves that the need for regulation outweighs our right to be let alone. We respectfully submit that the use of marihuana does not present such a clear and present danger, and that people have a constitutionally protected right to smoke marihuana if they so desire, in their pursuit of happiness."[619] When people do no harm they should not be harmfully punished. Such harmful behaviour is characteristic of arrogant bullies.

Peoples' prominent legal rights advocating: life, liberty, security, happiness and joy are cherished constitutional rights of fair and reasonable democracies, democracies intended to be *for* the people, by the people and of the people. Majority-vote rule is a prominent principle of constitutional democracies.

Governments should be helping people pursue their constitutional rights, not interfering, imposing or intruding into nonharmful private or personal affairs of people. "The right of people to be free from government intrusion into their private affairs is a right that we submit is guaranteed by the Constitution. The government may abridge this fundamental human right to be let alone, only if it demonstrates that there is a compelling interest to do so. . . . Society's interest in banning marihuana does not outweigh the right of people to use it, if they wish."[620] Improving one's life is a fundamental democratic right.

Despite confirmed medical abilities, natural and helpful green herb marijuana is still publicly unlawful and criminalized with secretively contrived man-made laws, while other man-made laws in our society allow people to harm themselves and others by drinking alcohol, a proven demonstrable harm maker. Such legal behaviour is inconsistent, unjust, discriminatory and unconstitutional, denying equal benefit of the law, and imposing harmful punishments on nonharmful people.

Man-made laws denying beneficial public uses of green herb marijuana also directly contravene another prominent democratic list of legal public rights, the Bill of Rights. More than one hundred years ago, in his classic essay 'On Liberty' John Stuart Mill (shown in a family picture below) explained that a government's exercise of its power over an individual is limited. He wrote, "The only purpose for which power can be rightfully exercised over any member of a civilized community, against his will is to prevent harm to others. . . . We submit that the guarantees found in the Bill of Rights and in the Fourteenth Amendment which forbid any state from depriving any person of life, liberty or property, without due process of law preserve to the

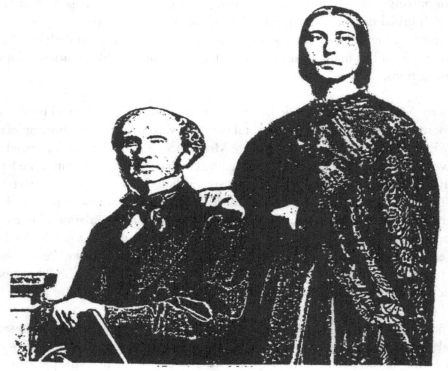

Footnote[621]

individual a right to privacy of thought and action."[622] "No society in which these liberties are not on the whole respected is free, whatever may be its form of government, and none is completely free in which they do not exist absolute and unqualified. The only freedom which deserves the name is that of pursuing our own good in our own way, so long as we do not attempt to deprive others' of their fair rights, or impede their nonharmful efforts. Each person is the proper guardian of his own health, whether body, mental or spiritual."[623] Essentially, liberty lawfully means doing whatever a person wants to do, providing no related truthful and demonstrabe harm is done to any person(s) or property.

Additional official U.S. court testimony concludes, "Marihuana is less dangerous to society than alcohol, and that the government in prohibiting one and not the other denies equal protection of the laws."[624] More U.S. court testimony under oath to tell the truth, the whole truth and nothing but the truth concludes, "As the LaGuardia Committee researchers found, marihuana quiets people and makes them more reflective. On the other hand, while alcohol may also quiet some people, it generally serves to weaken their inhibitions and may make them violent and unruly."[625] Although alcohol serves to weaken and destroy, while marijuana serves to heal and promote life and happiness, governmental laws discriminate against helpful marijuana plant participants, compared to government permission for people to drink harm-producing alcohol. Such obvious and true discrimination is contrary to principles of fundamental democratic justice.

Truthful and historic records exist. "In sum, it is clear that alcohol is more harmful to both society and the individual than is marihuana. And yet, while alcohol is a legal means for people to seek relaxation and enjoyment . . . marihuana is not. This arbitrary classification is without rational basis and unfairly discriminates against marihuana devotees. They have been denied equal protection of the laws guaranteed by the Fourteenth Amendment to the Constitution."[626]

Another substantiated report concludes, "The scientific evidence clearly demonstrates that marihuana is less dangerous than alcohol and therefore there is no rational reason to ban marihuana."[627] Similarly, "two government reports from the Le Dain Commission in the 1970s recommended decriminalization of possession" of marijuana.[628] Also, "the Canadian Bar Association adopted a policy supporting decriminalization of marijuana in 1976, including cultivation for personal use, and the nonprofit transfer of marijuana between people."[629] However, despite reasonable medical, scientific and moral recommendations, secretively-contrived criminal laws against nonharmfully using green herb marijuana plants remain in North America against God's directions.

Distrustful Harry Anslinger finally died in Pennsylvania on November 14, 1975. Perhaps it had something to do with, "his opium pipe collection."[630]

H. Anslinger and his clandestine cronies condoned hypocrisy. For many years, in bold print on U.S. paper currency have been the words, "In God We Trust". Yet Anslinger, a currency expert from the Treasury Department hypocritically denies trusting in God. When describing hypocrisy, a classic writer Alexander Pope explains, "Who dares think one thing and another tell my heart detests him as the gates of hell."[631] Although, Anslinger is now dead and gone, his harmful man-made criminal laws against God's green herb marijuana plants remain legally and hypocritically in effect.

The actual behaviour of prohibiting helpful uses of marijuana plants is religiously regarded as blasphemy against God. Hence, from a moral perspective alone, man-made laws against God's healthful marijuana should be eliminated before additional specific vengeance is meted out by God against those who promote punishing people for nonharmfully using God's preferred green herb marijuana plants.

It should often be remembered, when speaking to mortal people God said, "Behold, I have given you every herb. . . . to you it shall be for meat. . . . I have given every green herb for meat. . . . and thou shalt eat the herb of the field."[632] Blasphemy is detested by God. Mortal people supporting or promoting ideas contrary to God's directions is blasphemy.

On April 17, 1982 the Canadian Constitution Act was officially signed by Canada's Prime Minister Pierre E. Trudeau and Britain's Queen Elizabeth II. This act, "ended the need for British approval of amendments to Canada's constitution."[633] "Canada's bill of rights is called the Canadian Charter of Rights and Freedoms."[634] It was adopted as Part One of the Constitution Act in 1982. Section One of these current, most prominent laws in Canada declares, "The Canadian Charter of Rights and Freedoms guarantees the rights and freedoms set out in it subject only to such reasonable

By: Joseph W. Jacob B.A., M.P.A.

limits prescribed by law as can be demonstrably justified in a free and democratic society."[635] In other words, all laws in Canada are conditionally legally valid, subject to each of them first of all being truthfully, "demonstrably justified in a free and democratic society." Demonstrable justification requires *true* and *proven* harm to have been produced by the person *before* harmful punishment is imposed on that person. When people consume marijuana and no related harm is done, man-made laws against such actions and people cannot be demonstrably justified. Such laws then, against nonharmful public users of marijuana are not valid, because they are beyond the reasonable limits prescribed by law in a free and democratic society, as per Section One.

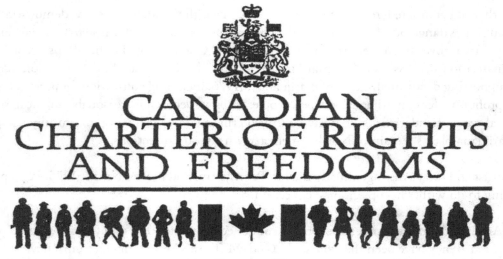

Footnote[636]

Also, 'guaranteeing' is essentially officially assuring the complete contents of all specific descriptions contained within this Charter of Rights and Freedoms. It has been demonstrably concluded in several substantiated studies that people drinking alcohol truthfully produce significantly more demonstrable harms than people who ingest marijuana. Therefore, logically and constitutionally marijuana should have a more favourable legal status in society than alcohol, because of alcohol's comparative harmful history. However, in true day-to-day Canadian actions, multi-harmful alcohol is legally available for public ingestion while multi-helpful green herb marijuana plants are not. This is *less than* equal benefit of the law and cannot be demonstrably justified in a free and democratic society, the multi-harmful product being given legal preference over the multi-helpful product. Constitutional fundamental justice is not truthfully demonstrated here. Discrimination is unlawful.

Section 7 of the Canadian Charter of Rights and Freedoms declares, "Everyone has the right to life, liberty and security of the person and the right not to be deprived thereof except in accordance with the principles of fundamental justice."[637] Principles of fundamental justice logically and morally prefer things that are beneficial and helpful, rather than things that are demonstrably harmful. Therefore, public marijuana laws should be much more favourable than society's alcohol drinking laws.

As per Sections 1 and 7(d) everyone is guaranteed the right to liberty which means doing anything that is not harmful. When a person does not produce true demonstrable harm(s) from ingesting marijuana, there is no justified and valid law in Canada against such people for using marijuana because demonstrable justification is legally *required* first.

The right to life is also denied to people who want to continue living or improve the health of their lives by medically using marijuana. Although people are dying from respiratory disorders, digestive difficulties, malignant cancers, depression, stress, AIDS, and a myriad of other harmful medical disorders, man-made laws do not allow nonharmful public citizens medical benefits from using helpful marijuana plants to improve their medically harmful conditions. Unjustified laws prohibiting nonharmful public uses of medically helpful marijuana plants do not guarantee actions advocating life, as described in Sections 1 and 7 of the Canadian Charter of Rights and Freedoms. This democratic right to life is also an important part of the U.S. Constitution where similar important democratic rights include: life, liberty and the pursuit of happiness.

In addition, as previously mentioned the important guaranteed right to liberty is being publicly denied. By not legally allowing beneficial public uses of God's helpful marijuana plants, valuable citizens are denied constructive pursuits in a 'free' and 'democratic' society. Freedom of choice to add value with no harm to people or property is the true legal essence of free enterprise democratic behaviour.

Another guaranteed fundamental charter right is: being presumed innocent until proven guilty, as described in Section 11 of the Canadian Charter of Rights and Freedoms.[638] The secretively-contrived and unprecedented North American man-made laws against marijuana users were enacted without substantiated, demonstrable and democratically proven truths. Little actual attention was shown for medically, scientifically, and behaviorly proving facts, so justified recommendations and democratic actions could be made. This fundamental democratic principle of being presumed innocent until truthfully proven guilty was never legally applied to the secretively contrived North American laws that suddenly publicly prohibited helpful uses of God's natural green herb marijuana plants.

As alluded to earlier, Section 15 of the Canadian Charter of Rights and Freedoms declares, "Every individual is equal before and under the law and has the right to the equal protection and equal benefit of the law without discrimination."[639]

Legally, each person is supposed to have "equal benefit of the law without discrimination." However, this is not the case with drinking alcohol as compared to consuming marijuana plants. Drinking alcohol has been demonstrated as actually producing considerably more true and factual harms in society than ingesting marijuana. Yet regarding discrimination, Canadian laws allow public consumption of harm-producing alcohol, but not of God's helpful and preferred marijuana plants. Healthful and versatile green herb marijuana plants are a part of improving life, whereas many reputable medical objective and scientific people have concluded that alcohol promotes death, because it is formed from decay and decomposition of dying organic (food) material. Such discriminatory laws are contrary to the Charter's principle guaranteeing equal benefit of the law.

Since the 1980s, nothing of a significant national legal change has occurred to eliminate this true discrimination factor between legalized public ingestion of harmful alcohol and legalized public ingestion of helpful marihuana. Alcohol is clearly known and demonstrated as truthfully producing significantly more actual demonstrable harms including social problems and medical disorders than do green herb marihuana plants. Yet, the harmful product alcohol remains legalized and promoted with man-made laws, while helpful and medically beneficial marihuana plants are not. "In fact, U.S. government police statistics confirm the following . . . numbers:

The mortality figures for alcohol use are 100,000 annually compared with zero marihuana deaths in 10,000 years of consumption.

From 40% to 50% of all murders and highway fatalities are alcohol related. In fact, highway fatalities that are alcohol related might be as high as 90% according to the Chicago Tribune and L.A. Herald Examiner.

Alcohol is also indicated in the majority (69% to 80%) of all child rape/incest cases, wife beating incidents are in the great majority (60% to 80%) alcohol influenced."[640]

Ingesting marihuana is also much safer than drinking alcohol. "Every U.S. Commission or federal judge who has studied the evidence has agreed that cannabis is one of the safest drugs known."[641] A related report concludes, "one of the most remarkable qualities of cannabis is its safety as a medicine. With a lethal to effective dose ratio estimated at 40,000 to 1, cannabis is far safer than Aspirin and most other legal medicines which commonly have a lethal dose only ten times greater than their effective one."[642] Hence, marihuana is truthfully thousands of times safer than medicines known to be lethal at only ten times their recommended dosage.

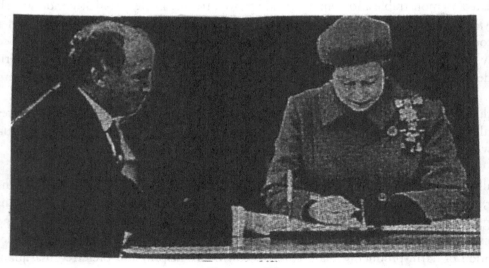

Footnote[643]

In 1982, official procedures were in progress to repatriate the Canadian Constitution from England and democratically authorize a new Canadian Charter of Rights and Freedoms. In April 1982, all sections of the Canadian Charter of Rights and Freedoms became legally and constitutionally approved. Sections 1 and 11(h) guarantee additional Charter protection to people convicted and punished for marijuana crimes. These two sections guarantee if a person is, "found guilty and punished for the offence not to be . . . punished for it again."[644] With typical current marijuana convictions, a person pays a monetary fine and/or a term of imprisonment. After that is completed, it is legally and constitutionally the end of the punishment, as per Sections 1 and 11(h). Oftentimes however, the person is punished again and again, particularly when trying to obtain a trustworthy job requiring 'bonding' for example, or international travelling. Peoples' careers are being ruined with families breaking-up, while poverties, stresses, miseries and depressions all increase. These and more harmful punishments occur for merely nonharmfully using God's helpful and preferred green herb marijuana plants. Such harmful legal behaviour is extremely unjust, contrary to the Citation section of the Canadian Charter of Rights and Freedoms legally describing Canada as a country that gives, "immeasurable joy". Legally expected then is a just and immeasurably joyful society.

Many respected, official, scientific international studies consistently conclude that ingesting marijuana is truthfully helpful rather than being demonstrably harmful. "Nearly 100 years have passed, since the 1894 British Raj Commission Study of hashish smokers in India reported cannabis use was harmless and even helpful. Numerous studies since have all agreed, the most prominent being: Siler, LaGuardia, Nixon's Shafer Commission, Canada's Le Dain Commission, and the California Research Advisory Commission."[645]

In 1980, Prime Minister Trudeau's federal government desired, "to move marijuana offences from the Narcotics Control Act to the Food and Drug Act to avoid criminal prosecution and jail terms."[646] By 1981, the Canadian Medical Association declared its stance that marijuana possession, "should not be a criminal offence."[647] In addition, a confidential discussion paper put out by the federal justice ministry under Jean Cretien, also in 1981 recommended the federal government, "ensure that the legal response to cannabis use does not result in unnecessary adverse consequences to individuals."[648] When no harm is first produced, *any* subsequent punishment(s) are 'unnecessary adverse consequences'. In truthful practise marijuana laws have produced violent demonstrable harms. Therefore, such laws are not legally and constitutionally valid because they cannot be demonstrably justified in a free and democratic society. Consider

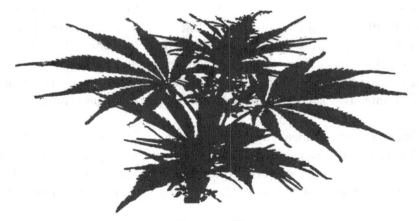

Footnote[649]

the following demonstrable harms produced by marijuana laws. An official Canadian Senate hearing reports, "police can even murder you in this country for smoking marijuana. . . . In 1991, the police shot dead in cold blood someone who merely had a few joints on them. It is certainly true in

Vancouver, when in 1992, a 16 year-old was shot dead by four North Vancouver police busting into his home for having merely a few joints."[650] Obviously, marijuana laws produce demonstrable harms including officials killing nonharmful defenseless citizens.

Similarly in March 2005, five people (four R.C.M.P. officers and one civilian) were murdered near a small Albertan community. The reason: police searching for marijuana plants. But, the plants did not produce the harms. It was laws with guns and bullets, and allowing their enforcement that actually and truthfully produced these deaths. When demonstrable harms are produced by man-made laws, such harmful laws cannot be "justified in a free and democratic society." When laws cannot be 'demonstrably justified' they are not constitutionally valid, as per Section 1 of the Canadian Charter of Rights and Freedoms.

Using marijuana is reconfirmed as being medically helpful for restoring appetites, such as with the medical disorder of anorexia nervosa. "Marijuana users often . . . get . . . a stimulated appetite for food which makes cannabis the very best medicine on the planet to date for anorexia."[651]

It is also concluded that ingestion of marijuana is good for reducing stress, which can cause: numerous nervous disorders, high blood pressure, premature old age, and mistakes (often harmful and sometimes deadly). It is reported, "Cannabis lowers blood pressure, dilates the arteries and reduces body temperature an average of ½ degree, thereby relieving stress. Even cannabis smokers in general report more restful sleep. Using cannabis allows most people a more complete rest with the highest among of 'alpha time' possible in sleep, as compared to prescription or sleep-inducing patent sedatives."[652]

A further impressive medical analysis about reducing stress by physically ingesting marijuana concludes, "Most of all, it is best for the world's number one killer stress. It can safely curtail or replace Valium, Librium or alcohol for millions of Americans."[653]

In addition, marijuana ingestion is medically beneficial for eyesight and vision. A published medical report of the 1990s describes, "Fourteen percent of all blindness in America is from glaucoma, a progressive loss of vision. Cannabis smoking would benefit 90% of our 2,500,000 glaucoma victims, and is two to three times as effective as any current medicines for reducing ocular pressure. And cannabis use has no toxic side effects to the liver and kidneys, nor is there any danger of the occasional sudden death syndromes associated with the legal pharmaceutical drugs/drops."[654]

Unlike alcohol and most commercially produced tobacco cigarettes currently manufactured and sold in North America, marijuana does *not* cause lung cancer. A significant medical report of the 90s concludes, "While tens of millions of Americans smoke pot regularly, cannabis has never caused a known case of lung cancer as of March 1992, according to American's foremost lung expert Dr. Donald Tashkin."[655]

Another official U.S. government study at about this time concludes that marijuana does not cause cancer. Near the beginning of 1997 in Massachusetts, "a $2 million dollar federal study which states that marihuana does not cause cancer has surfaced after being shelved for over two years. The

126

director of the National Toxicology Program explained that the delay in publicizing the study was because of a personnel shortage."[656]

When mentioning the many marvellous medical merits of multi-useful marijuana Mr. Gatewood Galbraith, candidate for Governor (State of Kentucky) concludes, "Hemp is the most beneficial plant that mankind has ever domesticated on this globe."[657]

Marijuana is also proving to be medically beneficial for people with AIDS, a harmful, serious and spreading current medical problem. "There are now 30 diseases listed under the condition known as Acquired Immune Deficiency Syndrome, AIDS. Most AIDS sufferers will contract several of these 30 during the course of their illness, before finally succumbing to one of them. The traditional medications used in both their treatment and as prophylaxis—or prevention—cause a wide range of side effects, including loss of appetite, nausea, headaches, depression, pain, disorientation and fevers. Virtually the only medicine capable of treating the entire spectrum of side effects without causing harm to the user is marijuana."[658]

A closely related harmful medical disorder is Human Immunodeficiency Virus (HIV). "A diagnosis of HIV+ changes to a diagnosis of AIDS when a patient either contracts one of the 30 AIDS diseases or when his or her T—cell count, representing the number of healthy immune cells the patient has falls below 200 (normal range is 800—1200). While most people believe that testing HIV positive is a death sentence . . . Greg Scott who tested positive for HIV in 1987 sees marihuana as a vital part of his treatment. My story actually begins with someone else's, he said recently. I watched a friend of mine, after he was told he was HIV positive give up all the things he enjoyed. He was a heavy drinker and he gave up drinking and he got healthier. He was a smoker and he gave up cigarettes and got healthier. But then he gave up marihuana and we noticed an immediate change. He stopped eating and was put on AZT, and the next thing you know he was losing weight. When I saw this, I realized that marihuana would play an important role in my therapy as my disease progressed. It's a key factor for me in terms of stress reduction, pain relief, eliminating nausea, and it gives me some degree of appetite. In fact, you could say I've devoted myself to smoking marihuana and eating good healthy food. "And I'm convinced that's what's keeping me alive at this point. I'm pretty healthy for someone with no immune system left. I just take a hit and feel immediately better."[659] Here's living proof of improving life with ingesting marihuana.

"Patrice . . . is a 36-year-old Colorado woman, who was diagnosed HIV+ nearly 10 years ago, and as an AIDS patient more than seven years ago, when her T-cells dropped to zero. She agrees with Scott on marihuana's importance. "I avoid their . . . therapies, smoke marihuana every day to maintain my appetite, and eat wholesome food. And if I feel low, I use natural herbs. The doctors just look at me, shake their heads and say, We don't know why you're the way you are, but whatever you're doing just keep doing it. . . .

As AIDS progresses and the medical therapies utilized intensify, marihuana also provides patients with help in easing joint and muscle pains, and reducing stomach cramps associated with morphine use. Additionally, marihuana use has been known to eliminate the drug-induced stupor suffered by many AIDS patients. . . .

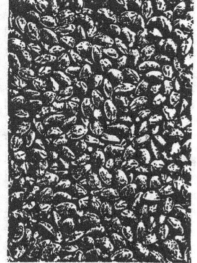

Footnote[660]

Mark Tildon, a 30-year-old wheelchair-bound hemophiliac from Washington state . . . contracted HIV from contaminated blood products. . . . Diagnosed HIV+ in 1988 Tildon had already discovered marihuana's medical benefits for relief of spasms in his hips.

As soon as I was diagnosed HIV+, I was put on AZT. It almost killed me. I was only on it for about two weeks, but I lost my appetite. The thing with HIV is you have the same loss of appetite whether you're on AZT or not. If I didn't have cannabis I would have starved to death a long time ago.

I take 255 pills every two weeks for pain and spasms, but the only thing that really works is the cannabis . . . something that works better and is natural."[661] Smoking, eating or drinking teas from marijuana leaves, buds and resins have shown positive medical results. Within the fertilized buds grow seeds, also reported as being very nutritious for human consumption.

A reliable medical report of the 90s explains, "Hemp seed can be pressed for its highly nutritious vegetable oil, which contains the highest amount of essential fatty acids in the plant kingdom. These essential oils are responsible for our immune responses, and clear the arteries of cholesterol and plaque. . . . Marijuana seed protein is one of mankind's finest, most complete and available-to-the-body vegetable proteins. Hemp seed is the most complete single food source for human nutrition."[662]

It is also recorded, "hemp seed contains 20% complete protein and about 30% oil. The sterile seed is legal to possess. . . . Hemp seeds are not psychoactive. A few pamphlets on cooking with hemp seeds are available."[663]

Other helpful medical uses of marijuana also became disclosed during the 1990s. "Even more important to building a strong immune system, hemp seeds are the highest source in the plant kingdom of essential fatty acids. These essential oils . . . are responsible for the luster in your skin, hair, eyes and even your thought processes. They lubricate (clear) the arteries and are vital to the immune system.

These essential fatty acids have been used . . . to successfully treat 'terminal' cancer patients, as well as those suffering from: cardiovascular disease, glandular atrophy, gall stones, kidney degeneration, acne, dry skin, menstrual problems and immune deficiency. . . .

Using marijuana also improves conditions for people with tuberculosis. Cannabis seed protein even allows a body with nutrition-blocking tuberculosis, or almost any other nutrition-blocking ailment to get maximum nourishment."[664] It is also scientifically concluded, "No other single plant source can compare with the nutritional value of hemp seeds. Both the complete protein and the essential oils contained in hemp seeds are in ideal ratios for human nutrition."[665]

"Hempseed foods taste great and will insure we get enough essential amino acids and essential fatty acids to build strong bodies and immune systems to maintain health and vitality."[666]

Marijuana ingestion including its seed oil, lightly rubbed on the skin is reconfirmed as being medically beneficial for arthritis, especially in areas such as: elbows, knees, wrists, ankles and hips. Using marijuana seed oil, "is said to ease the pressure and pain in the joints of arthritis sufferers."[667]

Oil from marijuana plant seeds, "has medicinal qualities stemming from its high content of Omega 3, Omega 6 and Omega 9 fatty acids. These components of hemp oil are known to be helpful in lowering cholesterol and lessening inflammatory conditions due to autoimmune diseases like rheumatoid arthritis. The usual dosage is one tablespoon or more per day."[668]

Marijuana seed oil has traditionally been medically helpful in salves for sore muscles and surface headaches. Beneficial oils from marijuana seeds, leaves and flowers, "can be made into salves or creams that can be applied for local pain, relief from muscle aches or inflamed joints. . . . Remedies often prescribed poultices made of marijuana for medical conditions such as rheumatism. Salves can also be applied . . . for headaches near the surface of the skin. Some people also use the salve for skin conditions such as psoriasis. . . . The best way to make these medicines is with a base of marijuana oil. . . . The oil can be applied directly to the skin."[669]

Eating marijuana plant leaves and buds is also medically reported for helping arthritis sufferers. "When eaten, marijuana has both analgesic and antiinflammatory effects. This can be helpful in both Osteo and Rheumatoid arthritis, when joints become swollen and painful."[670] In addition, it is recorded that eating marijuana, "is also more effective than smoking for painful conditions. When smoked marijuana does have some pain relieving qualities, but for the most

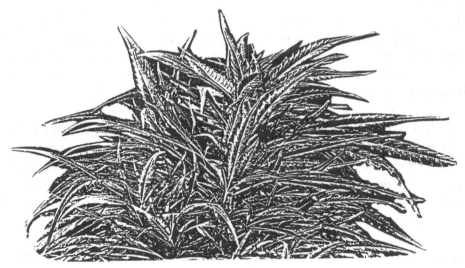

Footnote[671]

part these are related to relieving tension. When eaten however, cannabis has very strong analgesic and antiinflammatory effects."[672] This naturally relates to marijuana's traditional medical qualities of nourishing and healing peoples' organs and bodily functions. A vitally important related condition is, "people eating marijuana should refrain from using . . . alcohol."[673] Alcohol causes death. Marijuana bolsters life.

More recorded distinctions exist between eating and smoking marijuana. "There are some distinct differences both in the onset and in the duration of the high when marijuana is eaten. When pot is smoked the high comes on quickly, usually within ten minutes. It may take an hour or longer for the high to come on when marijuana is eaten. When smoked the high may last up to 3 hours, while when eaten the high can last 5 hours or more. Some of the medicinal effects can last up to 12 hours when the pot is eaten."[674] For thousands of consecutive years people have nutritiously enjoyed numerous types of marijuana foods. From cookies, candies and muffins to casseroles, sauces and teas, marijuana has been used in many traditional dishes and recipes. For monks in monasteries as well as workers in fields, people with pains, congestions, cancers and AIDS have nutritiously prepared and consumed healthy marijuana foods.

Another research statement of the 80s concludes, "(and it's still true in 1993) that after tens of millions of dollars and nine years of research on medical marijuana synthetics, "these drug companies are totally unsuccessful even though raw organic cannabis is a 'superior medicine' which works so well naturally on so many different illnesses."[675]

More research concludes that marijuana provides relief from herpes. "A separate study has shown that THC binds to the herpes virus and thus inactivates it. . . . Cannabis also provides symptomatic relief from gonorrhea and syphillis."[676]

In the United States, even the DEA (Drug Enforcement Agency) with its, "own conservative administrative law judge Francis Young . . . concluded in September, 1988 that marijuana is one of the safest therapeutically active substances known to man."[677] Living longer is another advantage attributed to ingesting marijuana. For most people living longer is an important medical benefit advocating the right to life. With international studies, "U.S. Costa Rican 1980-82, Jamaican studies 1968-74, statistical evidence . . . indicates that people who smoke tobacco cigarettes are usually better off and will life longer if they smoke cannabis moderately too."[678]

Similarly, "U.S. statistics indicate that you will live eight to 24 years longer if you substitute daily cannabis use, for daily tobacco and alcohol use."[679] Alcohol and intentionally contaminated cancer-causing commercial cigarettes are sending many more suffering citizens to earlier graves, than if people were legally allowed to use God's helpful, natural and preferred green herb marijuana plants. Not publicly allowing helpful medicine is a cruel, unusual and harm-producing crime against humanity.

It is similarly reported, "most studies (matched populations past and present) indicate that—everything else being equal—an average American pot smoker will live longer than his counterpart who does no drugs at all, with fewer wrinkles and generally less stress—thereby having fewer illnesses to upset the immune system, and being a more peaceful neighbor."[680]

Another important marijuana research observation of the 90s describes, "botanically, hemp is a member of the most advanced plant family on Earth."[681] Perhaps this is why it has so many favourable qualities.

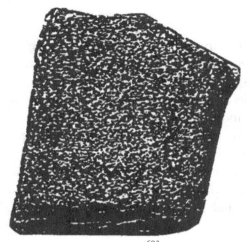
Footnote[683]

During the 1990s, even many old age pensioners were observed trying to obtain marijuana and hashish for healthful personal ingestion purposes. A related 1994 article in the Times of London explains, "The demand for cannabis among British pensioners has stunned doctors, police and suppliers. . . . The old people are using the drug to ease the pain of such ailments as arthritis and rheumatism. Many are running afoul of the law for the first time in their lives, as they try to obtain supplies."[682] Respect and medical help for elders is even denied with man-made marijuana laws. This is a callous sin against God's Fourth Commandment: 'Honour Thy Father And Thy Mother'. Disrespect and blasphemy violate God's laws, the most important laws of all.

Regarding reduction of public environmental deterioration and harms, marijuana legalization can also improve ozone damage to the earth, while increasing the world's supply of healthy oxygen. "Recent studies indicate that depletion of the ozone layer threatens to reduce world soya production by a substantial amount—up to 30% or even 50% depending on the fluctuation of the density of the ozone shield. But hemp, on the other hand resists the damage caused by increasing ultraviolet radiation, and actually flourishes in it by producing more cannabinoids which provide protection from ultraviolet light."[685] By allowing present trees and forests to continue growing and thereby providing a maximum amount of oxygen to the atmosphere, deforested or 'clear-cut' tree areas could also be cultivated with marijuana plants. This would continue to provide a substantial supply of construction materials and paper. In many areas, roads and bridges are already in place and closer to communities than expensively moving farther and farther away to dangerously remove more old growth oxygen factories (large trees).

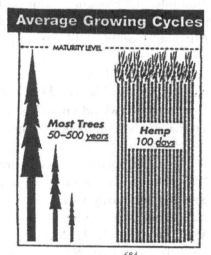
Footnote[684]

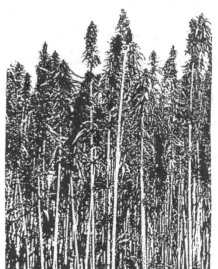
Footnote[686]

"Because one acre of hemp produces as much cellulose fiber pulp as 4.1 acres of trees, hemp is the perfect material to replace trees for pressed board, particle board, and for concrete construction moulds."[687] Also a mature marijuana crop can be grown in 90 to 120 days. Typical crops of mature hardwood or softwood trees need 50 to 500 years before reaching maturity. This is an average productivity difference of at least 150 crops to 1, on the same area of land, with lower operating costs.

"According to the U.S. Department of Agriculture, you can produce four times the amount of paper per annum from an acre of marijuana/cannabis/hemp than you can from an acre of trees, plus hemp paper production uses one-fifth the chemicals needed to process wood pulp. Hemp paper production would drastically reduce the need for clear cutting, and allow for reforestation to ensure the long term survival of not only the timber industry, but the life of our planet as well. . . . Hemp fabric is four times stronger than cotton, four times as water absorbant, and four times as soft. . . . Marijuana requires no pesticides . . . is a renewable crop, and the most effective plant for soil reclamation. Until 1915, marijuana was planted as ground cover and used to prevent mudslides and erosion."[688] This could be very valuable for improving land areas prone to harms from waters and winds, such as The Red River, Tornado Alley, Manitoba, Missouri, Mississippi, Alabama, Arkansas, Florida, and Lousianna.

Everyone in the world needs oxygen to breathe and live healthy lives. While the world's population rate is increasing, the world's rate of old growth, huge tree, oxygen factories is decreasing. Legislation *for* the people would encourage more supplies of life-giving oxygen available to its people, with alternate provisions of ample paper and construction supplies.

Marijuana plants are also more environmentally friendly than using petroleum fuels and trees. "Petroleum fuels are easily replaced by hemp-based fuels such as methanol, which is currently produced primarily with cornstalks. Hemp, however produces four times as much cellulose for making fuels like methanol than cornstalks do. . . . Most racing cars run on methanol. . . . The U.S. Army/Navy standards purchasing specifications list hemp oil as the number one preferred lubricant for their machinery."[689] North American farmers also stand to reap economic benefits from growing marijuana plants. One economic report concludes, "Farmers in Colorado estimate the per acre value of hemp at easily four times that of either corn or soybeans."[690]

"Farming 6% of the continental U.S. acreage with biomass crops would provide all of America's energy needs. Hemp is earth's number-one biomass resource, it is capable of producing 10 tons per acre in four months. Biomass can be converted to methane, methanol or gasoline at a cost comparable to petroleum, and hemp is much better for the environment. Hemp can produce 10 times more methanol than corn. Hemp fuel burns clean. Petroleum causes acid rain due to sulphur pollution. The use of hemp fuel does not contribute to global warming."[691]

Growing marijuana is also successful for removing weeds from soil, making the soil more suitable for cultivating other crops. This rare attribute typifies marijuana's many versatile values. "Almost any product that can be made from wood, cotton or petroleum (including plastics) can be made from hemp. There are more than 25,000 known uses for hemp. . . . Plastic plumbing pipe (PVC pipes) can be manufactured using renewable hemp cellulose as the chemical feed stocks, replacing non-renewable coal or petroleum based chemical feed stocks.[692]

Canada and the United States are perhaps seeing some dull glimmers of hope within the dank dismal darkness shrouding marijuana laws. During the spring of 1994, "Jim Kingston, executive director of the Canadian Police Association said he wants marijuana decriminalized."[693] Another report in 1995, titled 'War Without Winners' describes how the war on drugs is an expensive failure. B.C.'s Chief Coroner and RCMP officer for twenty-five years, Mr. Vince Cain concludes, "The war on drugs is a failure, an expensive failure. We should not be hiring more police. We should not be directing addicts into the courts. We should not be building more jails. Addicts don't need jails. They need care. What we have now is a system that's persecuting society's victims. In Cain's 110-page report . . . he challenges many of the assumptions that underline Canada's current drug policy. . . . The evidence of failure is everywhere. . . . 50,000 Canadians die each year from effects of the country's two major legal drugs—cigarettes and

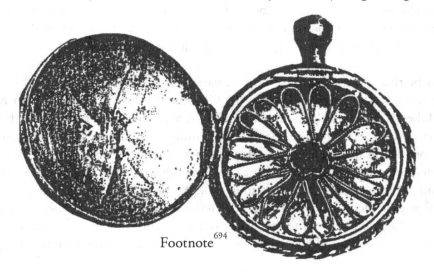

Footnote[694]

alcohol—while fewer than 1,000 die annually from all the illegal drugs combined. . . . A recent SFU study of coroners' reports indicate that of the 1,290 drug-overdose deaths in B.C. in the past decade, more than 50 percent were the result of people shooting up while blotto on booze."[695] Again, drinking alcohol results in more deaths.

In terms of logical, moral, economic and humane recommendations, Mr. Vince Cain, "calls for decriminalizing hard drugs and legalizing soft drugs like marijuana."[696]

Another sign of hope for legally publicly using marijuana appeared in Vancouver, B.C. A report on June 18, 1995, explains, "Simple drug possession in Vancouver will no longer be prosecuted under new federal government guidelines. . . . Senior federal drug prosecutor Mr. Lindsay Smith wrote to Vancouver police on May 17 advising them of the relaxed stance. . . . The edict applies to Vancouver, where drug prosecutions have overloaded the courts. . . . Vancouver police Deputy Chief Rich Rollins agrees. . . . "We have to be practical, that is the bottom line," Rollins said. He confirmed the letter had come after . . . meetings with federal justice department officials and drug prosecutors. . . . Prof. Neil Boyd, Head of Simon Fraser University's criminology department . . . advocates decriminalizing drug possession, saying drug use should not be a criminal offence. It doesn't make sense to criminalize the chemical alteration of consciousness with some drugs when we allow people to do it with tobacco and alcohol, Boyd said."[697]Life, logic, liberty, justice, joy, happiness, health and wealth would all be better served if marijuana plants once again become legally available for nonharmful public uses.

Has history taught us nothing? History is like a proficient compass, providing reliable guidance to a successful future. Results of prominent official marijuana research in Canada were published by the Le Dain Commission in 1972. Even this Commission, "recommended penalties for simple possession of marijuana and hashish be eliminated."[698] Justice delayed is justice denied. Stifling nonharmful initiatives is selfish, unjust, undemocratic, tyrannical and immoral.

In March 1996, "Canada's new Minister of Health introduced a motion that revived Bill C-7 the Controlled Drugs and Substances Act. The bill was renamed Bill C-8 and deemed passed by the House of Commons. Apart from changing the Bill's number from C-7 to C-8, this version of the Controlled Drugs and Substances Act was identical to the Bill originally passed by the House of Commons on October 30, 1995, the day of the Quebec referendum."[699] The entire Bloc Quebecois Party protested marijuana prohibition laws, by walking out of the House of Commons, en masse to avoid being part of condemning God's green herb marijuana plants even more.

"It used to be that it required consent of all parties in the House for a bill which died in this manner to be revived. This was changed by the Conservative government of Brian Mulroney. At the time, the Liberals complained about this 'undemocratic' change in process, but have now used the exact same procedure to get their legislation through without debate."[700] It's similar to the undemocratic procedure used during the dirty-thirties by Harry Anslinger and Andrew Mellon. Sidestepping democratic debates and majority-rule voting avoided presentations of the truth, the whole truth and nothing but the truth so help us God. By avoiding democratic public participation, it is reported that penalties for possession are not reduced, police powers of search and seizure are increased and the, "act will streamline the justice system to allow for more trafficking charges to be laid."[701] Justice for the people and by the people are not evident here where no harm is produced.

Some rays of democratic hope began glimmering from the United States during the 1990s. In 1992, San Francisco voters passed Proposition P, officially acknowledging, "a medical marijuana nonenforcement policy."[702] This made medical marijuana the lowest enforcement priority for city police. Two other nearby counties of Santa Cruz and Oakland soon passed similar resolutions.

By the mid 1990s, a new organization emerged in California encouraging Proposition 215, a statewide initiative for legalizing medical uses of marijuana. Californians for Compassionate Use began collecting enough appropriate signatures to have this public

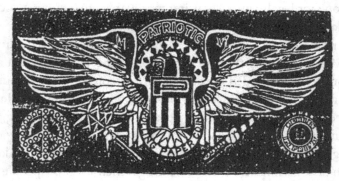

Footnote[703]

referendum issue democratically placed on their state's U.S. election ballots of November 1996. Dennis Peron, a marihuana crusader from San Francisco helped lead a campaign, "that collected

763,000 signatures to get Proposition 215 on the November 1996 ballot."[704] The Compassionate Use Act (Proposition 215) declares its primary purpose is to, "ensure that patients and their primary caregivers who obtain and use marihuana for medical purposes, upon the recommendation of a physician are not subject to criminal prosecution or sanction."[705] During this election campaign, "Yes on 215 announced the endorsement of . . . the California Academy of Family Physicians—with 7,000 doctors statewide . . . the San Francisco medical society . . . and the American Public Health Association . . . all registered support."[706]

Results from 1996 U.S. elections in California and Arizona showed majority-vote support for medical uses of marihuana. Majority-vote rule is a prominent principle of democratic fundamental justice. Harmful behaviour by the U.S. federal government against these new laws would probably, "escalate the debate now sweeping America over the powers of states versus the federal government."[707] On December 30, 1997 the U.S. federal government announced, "its plan to oppose implementation of Proposition 215 by threatening California doctors with a wide range of punishments if they recommend medical marihuana."[708] In response, "a group of physicians and patients filed a class action suit in federal court, in San Francisco seeking an injunction to prevent federal officials from taking any punitive action against physicians who recommend the medical use of marihuana to their patients in compliance with California law."[709] In court, Judge David A. Garcia ruled in favour of medical uses of marihuana. His reasoning was based on what he called, "the will of the people as shown by 56% of California voters passing the Compassionate Use Act (Proposition 215) on November 5, 1996."[710] In our growing democratic world perhaps public sentiment may lean in favour of supporting more free choice marijuana propositions placed on governments'

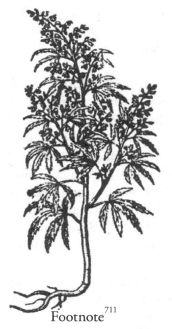

Footnote[711]

election ballots. California, Maine, Nevada, Washington State, Arizona and Alaska are providing responsible leadership in democracy for the people, by the people and of the people. From 1996 to 2000 each of these seven states legally voted in democratic public election referendums, all approving medical uses of marihuana. By 2005 four more states joined the same democratic course of action. In the U.S. elections of November 2008 the state of Michigan also voted approval for medical uses of marihuana. In addition, the state of Massachusetts voted and approved decriminalization of marijuana, replacing it with monetary fines starting at $100 per infraction for possessing one ounce or less of marihuana. An important intention is to avoid criminal records for nonharmful people who possess small amounts of marihuana. A related Harvard University study estimates an annual saving of $30 million in reduced policing costs alone for the state of Massachusetts. The will of the majority legally prevailed. In the U.S., marihuana issues may be decided by the people voting. But in Canada, no referendum has ever been legally conducted to approve medical or nonharmful uses of marijuana.

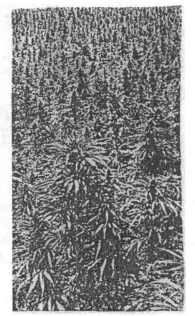

Footnote[712]

By: Joseph W. Jacob B.A., M.P.A.

In 1982, Canada's national anthem received lawful recognition as being part of the Canadian Constitution. A country's national anthem typically summarizes legal aspirations of its people and their governments. In this national anthem, 'Oh Canada' are the words 'Glorious and Free' and 'the True North Strong and Free'. Freedom is not evident when the public is denied legal access to nonharmful or medical uses of marijuana. However, more legal corrections may develop. In 1996, Canadian Senators showed sound leadership by trying to improve the future for God's marijuana plants. Represented by Senator Lorna Milne, an amendment was made to Bill C-8 making, "it legal to cultivate some forms of marijuana or hemp, by adding 'mature hemp stock' to a list of approved substances."[713] Senator Milne advised, "It seems to me to be a sensible thing to do."[714] Similarly, "Environmentalists say a domestic hemp industry could reduce destructive logging practices, by replacing wood-based pulp in the paper making process. . . . Hemp activists . . . welcome the news that Canada may soon be able to compete in the world hemp market."[715] Geoff Kime, business director of 'Hempline' added, "under NAFTA hemp can be exported to the U.S. duty-free."[716]

In June 1996 the Canadian Federal House of Commons officially approved Bill C-8, a good-news, bad-news set of laws. The cultivation and sale of hemp plant stock received approval, "by Parliament."[717] But possession of marijuana buds, leaves, and resins (hashish) remained a criminal offence. With mature hemp stock now legalized, courageous Senate leader Lorna Milne concludes, "It is bound to create jobs in the agriculture industry, as well as spinoffs and economic activity related to its products."[718] However, with this new Canadian man-made law, even dirt in Canada receives legal preference over the public regarding medical uses of marijuana. "While the stock and seeds are commercial products, the leaves where the THC accumulates are a controlled substance and must be stripped from the plant and turned into the soil, before the crop can leave the farm."[719] So, even soil on the farm has legal preference over the general Canadian public for medical uses of marijuana. When soil receives preference over people, there could be flaws with the laws. Discrimination contravenes democratic principles of fundamental justice. Guaranteed rights of liberty and equal benefit of the law are in sections 1, 7 and 15 of the Canadian Charter of Rights and Freedoms. In Canada's democracy,

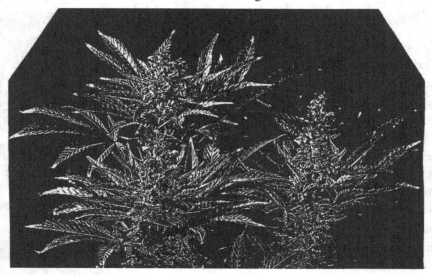

Footnote[720]

everyone who does no harm is guaranteed the right and freedom of liberty, freedom of choice to improve their lives. When such people choose to medically improve themselves by nonharmfully using marijuana leaves, buds, seeds or resins, that is their guaranteed constitutional right of liberty as well as their guaranteed legal right to "equal benefit of the law".[721] According to the original Bible, people are supposed to have dominion over everything on earth including soil. Therefore, preference should be with people, each person to choose their nonharmful involvement with marijuana use(s).

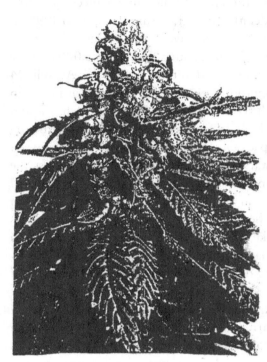

Footnote[725]

During 1997, the B.C. Ministry of Agriculture encouraged cultivating more cannabis plants. Agriculture Minister, Mr. Evans, "sees hemp production as a case of 'everybody wins'. It's an excellent niche crop and a source for more agricultural business. The Agriculture ministry wants Ottawa to lift its restrictions on growing hemp."[722] An experienced cannabis farmer who has legally cultivated hemp plants under federal licence for several years, recently explained that British Columbia, "is best suited for seed production rather than fibre production."[723] Along with the B.C. Ministry of Agriculture, other significant organizations have also supported legalization of marijuana plants. The Bank of Montreal and Environment Canada have similar supportive attitudes as those from the B.C. Ministry of Agriculture. In early 1996 for example, more than 250 people attended a conference on industrial hemp in Toronto. "The two-day event was no counter-culture clambake. Its sponsors included the Bank of Montreal and Environment Canada."[724] A spokesman for the Bank of Montreal, Peter Brown explains, "We recognize the value of this potential emerging market which will support Canadian agriculture and farmers."[726] Some farmers in eastern Canada received authorization to cultivate cannabis plants before 1997. In 1994 for example, Canada's first legal marijuana plant crop, "since the 1930s was harvested under a special research licence and under the watchful eyes of the RCMP."[727] Then, with approval from the Canadian federal controlled Substances and Abuse Act, in June 1996 more licences were issued to other Canadian farmers. "This new legislation permits farmers to cultivate and sell industrial hemp, the nonnarcotic form of Cannabis Sativa."[728] 1997-1998 saw more applications for commercially cultivating hemp plants being approved by Health Canada. In June 1997, Ottawa issued a licence to the Granby Hemp Co-op on Vancouver Island in B.C., "to grow 11 ½ hectares (28 acres) of hemp for oil. It is the first licence issued in B.C."[729] The small and healthful community of Grand Forks in southern B.C., also received a federal licence to commercially grow hemp plants. In June 1997, a joyous report describes how Grand Forks is, "celebrating yesterdays arrival of a federal licence to grow 11.5 hectars of hemp, raise it to maturity and press the seeds for oil. A hemp-oil factory in Ohio will ship a press to make the oil."[730] In February 1998,

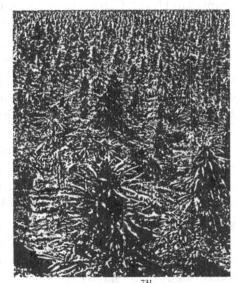

Footnote[731]

Canada's Health Minister (Honourable Allan Rock) approved procedures for legally cultivating hemp in Canada. "Canadian farmers can plan to grow hemp this spring for the first time in 60 years. Health Minister Allan Rock announced a quicker-than-expected green light for the crop, at the annual meeting of the Canadian Federation of Agriculture."[732] Also in 1998, at a symposium in Vancouver, a representative from Manitoba said, "We are looking forward to 2,000 or more acres (833 hectares) in Manitoba in 1998."[733] As well, 24 farmers in Ontario received approval to cultivate hemp plants through the University of Guelph, who has a pilot project, "in which 24 farmers are committed to growing two-hectare packages above the 50th parallel between Sudbury, Ontario and the Manitoba border to test the plants' hardiness to the northern growing season."[734] Another Ontario hemp business, Hempola, "plans on establishing a hemp-seed crushing plant in Manitoba this summer to take advantage of the new crops."[735] In March 1998, Canadian farmers, "applied for permits to grow 3,500 hectares of commercial hemp across Ontario and the Prairies."[736] Also in March 1998, Health Minister Allan Rock unveiled rules for cultivating hemp in Canada. He said, "Farmers . . . across the country have an opportunity to diversity their crops in a way that makes economic sense and in a way that's good for the environment."[738] As the current legal approving authority, "Health Canada licences producers of cannabis with flower heads containing no more than 0.3 percent THC."[739] Also, the Canadian federal government, "will control all activities relating to the plant's import, export and handling."[740] Canadian farmers who want to grow ten-acre plots of industrial hemp may now apply to Health Canada for legal approval to do so. "Thanks to recent changes in Health Canada regulations, farmers can now grow 10 acres of industrial hemp. . . . Hemp oil is proving to be the most nutritional oil."[741]

Footnote[737]

In July 1998, a Vancouver Island farmer received a permit from Health Canada to cultivate a crop of industrial hemp plants. One of his first requirements was to buy, "a global positioning system to determine the exact location of the authorized hemp farm."[742] Another related requirement was that he participate in a police check regarding his credibility.

Hemp plant production is realistically compared to being an, 'economic golden apple'. "It requires a minimum of chemical fertilizers and almost no pesticides to grow. It provides some of the most sturdy and durable fibres in nature—fibre that can create anything from clothes and paper to wallboard and car parts. . . . It's a soil builder. It's one of the crops that actually contributes to soil structure. It leaves the soil in better condition than when it started. . . . There are also few insects that have taken a shine to the crop leaving no need to spray it with chemical insecticides. . . . But hemp's main economic attributes come from the sturdy and versatile fibres it can provide to numerous industries. A main market attraction to hemp is the stock, because the stock yields several different types of fibres. These fibres have a reputation of having very unique exceptional qualities for strength and longevity. . . . It's also impervious to ultraviolet rays and is not like cotton or other plant fibres susceptible to mildew, so it doesn't rot. . . . Experts say about one hectare of hemp could produce the same quantity and quality of paper as 20 hectares of trees, leaving those trees to stand for future generations. Hemp's shorter fibres can also be crushed into building-board material, as well as auto accessories like dashboard padding and roof insulation. The plants seeds, on the other hand offer another range of possibilities. The seeds have the most nutritionally balanced oil of any vegetable oil."[743]

Legal changes improved development of low-level THC Canadian cannabis production. Good news was also concluded about consuming medically useful, or high-level THC cannabis plants. The more natural THC in marijuana plants, the more medically beneficial attributes are produced from such plants.

Plants with medically beneficial attributes are constitutionally allowed for each Canadian to consume. Improving one's life, without discrimination or harm is guaranteed to every person in Canada, as per Sections One, Seven and Fifteen of the Canadian Charter of Rights and Freedoms. Lawyer, Aaron Harnett recently testified in an official Ontario court, that laws against publicly using marijuana should be struck-down as unconstitutional. Regarding marijuana he said, "There has been renewed interest in its calming properties, since the outbreak of HIV. Tests have indicated that cancer chemotherapy patients have benefitted from marijuana's anti-nauseous qualities, he said. He testified it was much more effective to smoke the marijuana plant than to ingest the synthetic. He said there is no scientific study to show that marijuana will kill, or cause emphysema, memory loss, lung cancer, or lead to the use of other stronger drugs."[744] Recent scientific studies also conclude, "there is no difference between the marijuana user and nonuser in terms of willingness and ability to perform tasks, putting to rest the rumour that marijuana smokers are lazy."[745] Similarly, Dr. John Paul Morgan, a professor of pharmacology at City University of New York Medical School testified, "none of the drugs prescribed to epileptics is as safe as marihuana."[746]

More recently, Canadian laws against marijuana were declared 'unconstitutional'. In July 2000, Ontario's top official court gave, "the federal government a year to rewrite the law prohibiting possession. The law prohibiting possession of marijuana was declared unconstitutional . . . by Ontario's top court—a decision hailed by some as a step toward decriminalizing the drug across the country. In a unanimous decision, the Ontario Court of Appeal ruled the possession law violates Canada's Charter of Rights and Freedoms, because it fails to make exceptions for people who require marijuana for medicinal purposes. But rather than strike down the law outright, the court gave the federal government one year to rewrite its legislation to comply with the Charter. Possession will remain a criminal offence for 12 months, but if the government fails to act in that time the law will cease to exist and simple possession will become legal in Canada."[747] This case involves, "Terry Parker, a 44-year-old Toronto man who smokes marijuana to control his epilepsy. The judge had concluded and the Appeal Court agreed that Parker requires marijuana for health reasons, and that the possession law infringed his Charter rights. "I have concluded that forcing Parker to choose between his health and imprisonment violates his rights to liberty and security of the person, Justice Marc Rosenberg wrote in the Ontario Court of Appeal decision."[748]

A person who produces no harm should neither be harmed by police nor should the same person be harmed by the courts. The only people who should *not* be legally allowed to use marijuana are those who truthfully produce harm(s) as a result of consuming marijuana, and/or those who claim they produced harm(s) by using marijuana. Merely because some harmful criminals try obtaining reduced penalties by blaming marijuana does not justify imposition of harmful punishments on everyone else, by publicly prohibiting a helpful and safe medicine. Only true demonstrable harm-producers deserve punishments.

At this time, Ontario Superior Court Justice John McCart testified, "he was convinced marijuana was harmless and caused no serious mental or physical harm. But the judge ruled it would be up to Parliament to determine what's illegal."[749]

After the Ontario Superior Court court ruling in 2000, Vancouver City Police Constable Anne Drennan indicated support for public legalization by explaining, "Vancouver police rarely process possession of marijuana charges."[750]

Also, the Canadian federal government began encouraging protection for ill Canadians with degenerative health diseases. In 1999-2000, Health Minister Allan Rock started awarding, "special exemptions to some ill Canadians who can prove they need to smoke marijuana to control diseases such as AIDS and cancer."[751] In July 2001, Canada became, "the first country in the world to legalize the use of marijuana for medical purposes."[752] On this momentous occasion, the Canadian federal government enacted, "Medical Marijuana Access Regulations to comply with the [Terry Parker] decision."[753]

In September 2002, a Canadian federal government senate committee reached a similar ethical conclusion, "Marijuana, their final report concluded should not just be decriminalized and subject to petty fines but legalized altogether."[754]

In the United States, another removal of public medical nutrition occured during 2002. Without public approval, the Drug Enforcement Agency (DEA), "ordered any food containing hemp off store shelves. . . . This is from the same administration that says it's OK to have more arsenic in water."[755] An erosion of public nutritional rights and freedoms occurs with each unjustified legal restriction or removal of healthy (biologically electron rich) food. Beneficial and nonharmful foods and medicines should always be readily available *for* the people.

The Canadian legal approach continued changing in 2003. An, "Ontario judge ruled Canada's law on possession of small amounts of marijuana is no longer valid dismissed charges against a Windsor Ont., youth."[756] A Toronto lawyer testified in court, "The government has been overstepping its legal authority for the last 80 years by keeping a law on the books that provides for jail terms in simple possession cases."[757] In June 2003, "Toronto police Chief Julian Fantino told officers to stop laying charges for simple possession of marijuana."[758] A spokesperson said, "Obviously our political leaders are going to have to address this issue head-on and tell Canadians just where they stand on possession of marijuana."[759]

The Canadian legal climate suddenly changed in the fall and winter of 2003. On October 7th, the Ontario Court of Appeal declared, "Canada's law against possession in effect."[760] This meant marijuana possession in Canada was officially illegal, once again. No truthful demonstrable justification or harmful medical explanation was given. Similarly, in December 2003 the Supreme Court of Canada upheld a federal law prohibiting possession of small amounts of marijuana. "It's up to parliament to decriminalize the drug, says the 82 page ruling."[761] Again, contrary to Section 1 of the Canadian Charter of Rights and Freedoms, *no* truthful demonstrable explanation, or proven harmful evidence was provided by the court for justifying this ruling.

Hints of hope have been expressed by some Canadian politicians. Paul Martin, "has said in the past that he favours decriminalization in principle."[762] In 2004, Mr. Martin also said, "he intends to soon reintroduce a bill—first proposed by his predecessor Jean Cretien—to decriminalize possession of small amounts of cannabis in Canada."[763]

In 2004, Bill C-10 was introduced in the House of Commons. It would make possession of up to 15 grams of marijuana, "and up to three marijuana plants punishable by tickets and fines of $100-$500."[764] Scales of fundamental justice are *not* in balance when the amount of harmful punishment imposed exceeds the amount of truthful harm produced. When no related harm is produced, no harmful punishment is valid. 0 and $100 to $500 are far from being equal.

Canada and the U.S. are developing different legal environments regarding medical uses of marijuana. The U.S. federal government seems rather reluctant in allowing helpful public uses of marihuana plants. One report in 2005 concludes that some influential members of the U.S. federal government have, "made it clear that they wish to eradicate cannabis and hemp plants from the face of the earth. It's not because these plants pose any real danger to the users or society, but because they are a danger to the oil-based economic wealth."[765] But, competition is a fundamental principle of free enterprise democracies. Competition typically improves values and lowers costs to consumers.

More locally in the U.S., several states have approved medical uses of marijuana using official majority-rule democratic referendum voting. In 2005, it is reported there are now, "eleven U.S. states . . . and over 100,000 legally registered medical marihuana users in the state of California alone, compared to Canada's roughly 850."[766]

Canadian attitudes may become more caring and humane. One report during 2005 explains, "Vancouver City Council is pressing for legalization of marijuana, while Parliament is considering legislation to remove criminal penalties for possession of small amounts."[767]

Improving peoples' health is beneficial both to the person and to society. Healthy people typically have abilities and ambitions to add more value, be more joyful and incur less hospitalization costs than unhealthy unproductive people. Publicly prohibiting or unjustifiably restricting a helpful medicine are crimes against humanity, contrary to principles of fundamental justice, principles providing nonharmful public legal rights advocating: life, liberty, happiness, joy, security, protection, equal benefit of the law, and truthfully proven harm *preceding* punishment.

CONCLUSION

YEARNING FOR THE WAY
IT USED TO BE

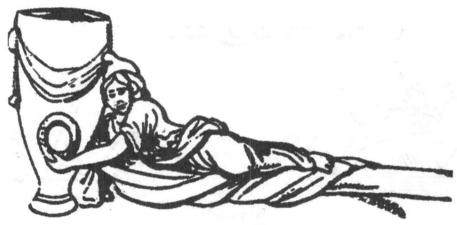

Footnote[768]

Throughout history many areas around the world have enjoyed numerous medical uses of marijuana. Among the traditionally recorded places include: China, India. Arabia, Assyria, Persia, Phoenicia, Africa, Afganistan, Pakistan, Burma, Russia, Japan, Romania, Bulgaria, Lithuania, Korea, Israel, Czechoslovakia, Yugoslavia, Jamaica, South America, Australia, Canada, the United States, England, Scotland, Wales, Ireland, Holland, Poland, Iran, Iraq, Italy, France, Germany, Greece, Hungary, Palestine, the Philippines, Mexico, Spain, Sweden, Switzerland, Tibet and Turkey. The sum of these geographic areas includes most of the land masses and human populations on earth.

Marijuana plants were initially intended for the medical benefit of everyone, including ordinary people represented by the pipe below, along with all other more priveleged people represented by the crown. The greatest good for the greatest number, or the greatest good for the largest amount of people became respected and traditional practices with using natural marijuana plants for improving health, wealth, security and surroundings of those involved.

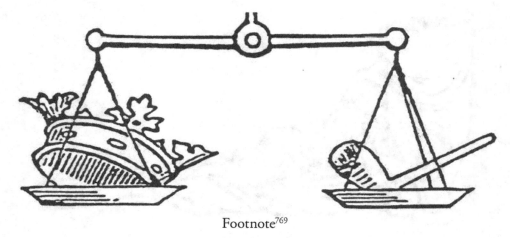

Footnote[769]

More than 150 different successful medical uses have been identified and confirmed with publicly ingesting green herb marijuana plants during the last 10,000 years of world history. Marijuana plants are recorded as being medically helpful for reducing: mental depression, pain, anxiety, stress, excessive coughing, gastrointestinal cramps, infantile convulsions, menstrual cramps, labor pains (and difficulties with childbirth), high blood pressure, spasmodic coughs, convulsions, absentmindedness, inflammation, earaches, menstrual fatigue, bladder irritations, mental confusion and migraine headaches.

Marijuana is also recorded as being medically helpful for improving: arthritis, rheumatism, speach, alertness, bronchitis, blood poisoning, constipation, gastric ulcers, diarrhea, epilepsy, contractions during childbirth, tetanus, malaria, lockjaw, teeth problems, anthrax, beri-beri, cholera, menorrhagia, palsy, rabies, senile insomnia and strychnine poisoning.

In addition, marijuana plants are recorded as being medically useful for quickening digestion and increasing mental powers,

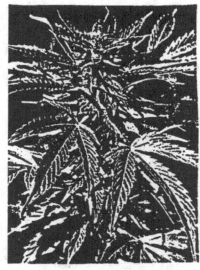

Footnote[770]

as well as for curing: fevers, sunstroke, ear problems, coughs, jaundice, leprosy, dysentery, stomach ailments, hemorrhoids, polyps of the throat, polyps of the intestines, and addictions from morphine and chloral-hydrate. Marijuana use is also medically recorded for correcting: irregularities of the phlegmatic humor, in addition to easing: cholic, pains of gout, pains of the hips, blackwater fever, sciatica, swelling of the liver, tic douloureux, and withdrawal symptoms from morphine and alcohol. Trusted medical documents report on successful uses of marijuana plants for healing: burns, injuries, waste-diseases, respiratory disorders and whooping cough. Marijuana plants are also recorded as being medically useful for relieving: AIDS, asthma, headaches, tension, herpes, fatigue, psychosis, seizures, syphillis, hysteria, delerium tremens, acute mania, insanity and nervousness, as well as for: stopping nose bleeds, dissolving harmful deposits in bodily joints, dressing wounds, drying up tumors, clearing blood, checking discharges from gonorrhea, lowering intraocular pressure in glaucoma, and calming spasms.

Additional encouraging records describe medical uses of marijuana for promoting: mental cheerfulness, internal heat, staying power, discharges of pus, astringency (reducing the size of a body canal) and a sense of well-being. More documents describe marijuana's medical usefulness for removing: dandruff, phlegm, wind (digestive gases) and vermin from people. Other medical uses of marijuana plant goods are reported to include: managing cancer and arousing appetites, as well as for helping with: Parkinson's Disease, muscular dystrophy, multiple sclerosis, osteo arthritis, rheumatoid arthritis, psoriasis, melancholy, nausea from chemotherapy, obsessive compulsiveness, inability to sleep (insomnia), saving people from attacks of evil influences, stopping children from crying, and putting women in happy moods.

More records describe healthful uses of marijuana as a: muscle relaxant, analgesic, sedative, anesthetic (such as in surgical anesthesia) and anti-convulsant, as well as being a solace in discomfort, and a cure in sickness. Trusted medical documents also describe nourishing uses of marijuana plants for improving tuberculosis, and for combatting: loss of memory and aging. In addition, marijuana has been medically useful for successfully treating, "terminal cancer patients."[771]

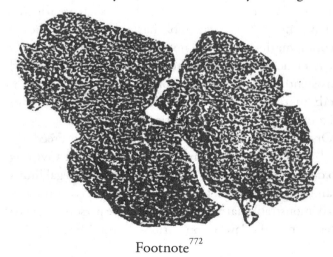

Footnote[772]

Other valuable medical treatments with using marijuana plant components have been for: gall stones, kidney degeneration, tumors, acne, alcoholism, glandular atrophy, cardiovascular disease, dry skin, snakebites, spider bites, parasites, immune deficiency, incontinence, uterine hemmorrhage, relieving back spasms, and for developing healthy lusters to skin, hair and eyes. More impressive medical uses of marijuana have been for improving: peptic ulcers, gastritis, dysmenorrhea, colitis, ileitis, mastitis, spastic colon, menstrual and postpartum pains, and to increase lactation. Just listed are more than 150 different beneficial medical uses of marijuana, that have been identified and recorded throughout history. In addition, many other choice quality products from marijuana plants have also been produced. Among them are: foods, clothes, shelters, shoes, bedding, nets, ropes, bagging, paints, papers, art canvases, caulking, twine, windmill sails, covers for pioneer wagons, sails for ships, flags, currency, fine napkins, bird seed, altar cloths and for anointing kings, as well as for improving soils and being environmentally friendly.

Regarding the truth, the whole truth, and nothing but the truth so help us God, a most important truth is that marijuana is *not* a true narcotic because it truthfully does *not* have *any* of the demonstrably harmful characteristics of true narcotics.

1. Marijuana use does not produce headaches as do true narcotics. Controlled studies have shown marijuana ingestion successfully relieves headaches even migraines.
2. Marijuana use does not produce loss of appetite as do true narcotics. In fact, marijuana has restored many appetites.
3. Marijuana use does not inactivate internal bodily functions as do true narcotics.
4. Marijuana use does not cause people to stagger or fall as do true narcotics.
5. Marijuana use does not produce nausea as do true narcotics such as morphine or alcohol.
6. Marijuana use does not harm internal body organs including livers, lungs, and hearts (as do true narcotics).
7. Marijuana use does not produce tolerance, as do true narcotics. That is, more of the product is not needed each time to produce the desired result.
8. Marijuana use does not produce constipation as do true narcotics.
9. Marijuana use has no painful withdrawal symptoms as do true and harmful narcotics.
10. Marijuana use has not produced even one death throughout recorded history, whereas true narcotics have produced millions of substantiated deaths.

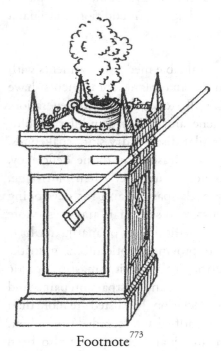

Footnote[773]

A primary purpose of democratic courts is to obtain and provide the truth, the whole truth, and nothing but the truth so help us God. A truth of the matter is that because marijuana does not have any of the demonstrably harmful characteristics of true narcotics, marijuana should not be unjustly and incorrectly classified as a true narcotic. Many nations throughout the world have consistently reported that publicly using God's natural green herb marijuana plants have truthfully improved lives *for* numerous people in many societies including democracies. Section One of the Canadian Charter of Rights and Freedoms for example guarantees that no law validly exists against anything where no demonstrable harm is done. It is *beyond* the legal limits in a free and democratic society to impose harmful punishments where no demonstrable harm is first done by the person. In short: no true harm, no valid law; or no harm—no punishment.

Marijuana plant seeds also promote the constitutionally guaranteed democratic right to life. Seeds from marijuana plants are nature's healthiest and most nutritious single food for human consumption. Also, no other plant source provides complete protein nutrition in such an easily digestible form. In addition, marijuana seeds contain all the essential amino acids and fatty acids necessary to maintain healthy human lives. These essential acids help improve our immune systems to avoid diseases such as AIDS. Foods that don't have biologically healthy electrons produce cancers in human bodies. However unlike most foods, eating marijuana seeds helps human body cells become biologically electron rich, which improves vitality for human bodies and allows them to live longer

and be stronger. This promotes the guaranteed democratic right to life as described in Section 7 of the Canadian Charter of Rights and Freedoms. Eating marijuana seeds also improves growth of body muscle fibres, in addition to reducing fat and plaque from clogging in human arteries. Similarly, these additional medical benefits promote our constitutionally guaranteed democratic rights to life, liberty and security of the person. Marijuana seeds are not psychoactive and they do not produce any demonstrable harmful effects (physical or mental). Seeds from marijuana plants are also devoid of narcotic effects. From the earliest times marijuana plants were prized, especially because of their abundance of nutritious seeds. "And God said, Let the Earth bring forth the herb yeilding seed and it was so, and God saw that it was good." Ingesting marijuana seeds became successful medical recommendations for: nervous disorders, convulsions, constipation, menstrual cramps and difficult childbirths. Respected ancient leaders used marijuana seeds for remaining strong, fertile and vigorous. Dioscorides, a famous and humane doctor who lived near

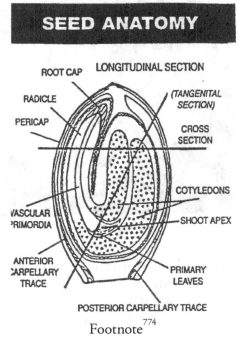

Footnote[774]

the time of Christ recommended marijuana seeds, in the form of a cataplasm to soothe inflammation. Similarly in the first century, Pliny the Elder of Rome describes that eating marijuana seeds produces medical improvements in treatments for: arthritis, gout and illnesses with similar symptoms. During the second century in Rome, eating marijuana seeds became medically recommended for relieving: poisoning, constipation and obstinate vomiting.

In Europe, dedicated religious monks have been required to eat marijuana seed meals three times a day, and to print their bibles on paper made with marijuana plant fibers. Also, respectful funeral rites have included obtaining purification with vapours from marijuana seeds. Near the beginning of the 1700s, the New London Dispensatory wrote that marijuana seeds were being medically helpful with treatments for: ulcers, sores, incontinence, and venerial diseases.

Even Samuel de Champlain, Father of new Canada brought Europeon marijuana seeds to the new colony. Seeds from marijuana plants became successfully grown in Port Royal, under the watchful eye of Canada's most prominent botonist and apothecary Louis Hebert. Diaries by Louis Hebert, "show he grew cannabis for his medical preparations."[775]

Canada's first Finance Minister Jean Talon legally supplied many Canadian farmers with marijuana seeds. In 1790, government officials of Canada co-ordinated delivery of two thousand bushels of marijuana seeds, that were distributed free of charge to all agricultural districts. President George Washington recommended to make the most of marijuana seeds and to plant them everywhere. He also had a marijuana plant farm. Another respected U.S. president Thomas Jefferson obtained rare marijuana seeds from Europe for American farmers. President Jefferson describes how hemp plants are of the first necessity to the wealth and protection of the country. In addition, oil from marijuana seeds lit lamps of Abraham the Prophet and Abraham Lincoln. It was the brightest lamp oil.

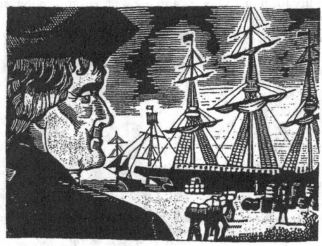

Footnote[776]

During the 1800s, marijuana seeds became popularly eaten for obtaining firm flesh and for prolonging lives of people. In addition, marijuana seeds were harvested as major cereal crops, along with barley, soybean, rice and millet. Marijuana seeds were also medically ingested for alleviating rheumatism and fevers.

Additionally, seeds from marijuana plants have been ground into pastes like peanut butter, but more flavourful. And there is more nutritional value in marijuana seeds than in typical peanut butters. Ground-up marijuana seeds and buds can be baked in breads, cakes, cookies, muffins, soups, casseroles and desserts. In the good old days, those who ate marijuana seeds became more resistant to disease. Eating marijuana seeds also reduces harmful cholesterol and plaque in human bodies.

Consuming marijuana seeds is biologically healthier than eating seeds from sunflower, sesame, flax and safflower. This is because only marijuana seeds contain gamma linolenic acid, an essential fatty acid not found in sunflower, sesame, flax, safflower and other common seeds. Furthermore, eating marijuana seeds has the capacity to cure neurological impairments due to stroke and the problems of excessive sweating which it brings on.

Recent studies have observed and concluded that when marijuana seeds are eaten for five to eight weeks by people with high blood pressure, such blood pressure is reduced and this medical treatment has no harmful side effects.

In addition, marijuana seeds have become medically beneficial for improving skin disorders including psoriasis.

Another trusted medical report about people eating marijuana plant leaves and tops including seeds concludes it is helpful for arthritis sufferers. When eaten, marijuana has both analgesic and anti-inflammatory effects, which can be helpful in both Osteo and Rheumatoid arthritis. In addition to building a strong immune system, marijuana seeds are the highest source in the plant kingdom of essential fatty acids which improve lusters in skin, hair and eyes. Eating marijuana seeds also lubricates and clears arteries of plaque. Furthermore, these essential fatty acids have been successfully used for treating terminal cancer patients, as well as for those suffering from: cardiovascular disease, glandular atrophy, gall stones, kidney degeneration, menstrual problems, dry skin and acne.

Protein from marijuana seeds even allows a body with nutrition-blocking tuberculosis and almost any other nutrition-blocking ailment to get maximum nutrition. Also, marijuana food products taste great and can ensure we obtain enough essential amino acids and fatty acids for building strong bodies and immune systems. This improves health, while exercising our democratic rights to: life, liberty, protection and security of the person. In terms of healthfully improving human lives, no other single food source can compare with the nutritional value of marijuana seeds. They are the single most nutritional food source for human consumption in the world. Perhaps this is a good reason why God prefers marijuana plants and their aromatic components.

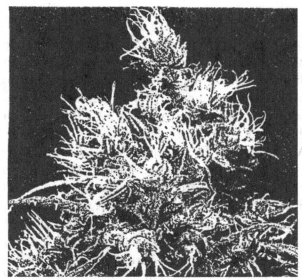

Footnote[777]

The prominent and primary purpose of democratic laws is to protect people and property from harm. This idea was espoused by fathers of democratic philosophy such as John Stuart Mill in his book, 'On Liberty'. Jeremy Bentham, another founding father of democratic philosophy championed the idea of 'the greatest good for the greatest number' of people. These and other pioneers of participative democracy held the belief that overall happiness and joy in society is found by legally allowing actions that improve both society and the individual person. When value is added everyone benefits. Similarly, democratic laws were approved to avoid harmful actions both to the person and to society, including related property. This is why so many medical uses of marijuana progressively developed, improving living standards both *for* society and *for* its individuals.

Also, democratic justice developed with an important legal purpose of providing the truth, the whole truth, and nothing but the truth so help us God. A truth of the matter is that marijuana does not have any of the harmful characteristics of true narcotics. Therefore, it should not be incorrectly legally classified to the detrimental health of humanity in general.

On the time spectrum of human history, this was an unexpected and unprecidented recent event. At no previous time in the annals of recorded history, for the past ten thousand years had any democratic government refused public access to medical and other helpful uses of marijuana plants. Afterall, marijuana herb plants were put on earth by God to improve lives of those choosing to participate. It wasn't until recently that secretive actions by democratic governments refused public legal access to medical uses of marijuana. The first time: 1923; the country: Canada. And no medical explanation or justification was legally provided. Nor were public Canadian citizens allowed to vote for this critically important legal change. It is still mysterious, "as to why marijuana was added— seemingly at the last minute and with almost no paper trail—to a list of drugs outlawed by the federal government in 1923. But most scholars believe that Emily Murphy's book prompted the ban."[778] A

By: Joseph W. Jacob B.A., M.P.A.

Canadian lawyer concludes that Emily Murphy, "was probably single-handedly responsible for the demonization—and the criminal convictions—of hundreds of thousands of Canadians over the years. Her writings were profoundly racist—a very, very vitriolic racist diatribe that had absolutely no basis whatsoever in science."[779] Perhaps Murphy's law contributed to this sudden unjust misclassification. Things were going fine until Emily Murphy and Mackenzie King got involved. And if things could go wrong they indeed did. Ultimately, most of the world's population would become harmfully affected by not being allowed legal public access to more than 150 different medical benefits provided by natural marijuana plants.

Throughout history, millions of people have obtained medical benefits from physically ingesting marijuana plant goods. Millions of others have suffered severely from the more than 150 different medical harms produced by drinking alcohol. In the process, many respected people and organizations participated in encouraging helpful uses of marijuana plant components, or denounced harm-producing alcohol-drinking. Included in this list are: Moses, Abraham, Aaron, King Soloman, Saint Paul, Jeremiah, Jesus Christ, Pythagoras, Nebuchadnezzar, Dioscordes, French Queen Arnegunde, President George Washington, President John Adams, Queen Elizabeth I, Queen Victoria, King James I, President Thomas Jefferson, Samuel de Champlain, Louis Hebert, Finance Minister Jean Talon, James Campbell, the Parliament of Canada, the General Court of Massachusetts, the General Assembly of Connecticut, the State of Virginia, the New London Dispensatory, Pilgrims, the New English Dispensatory, Daughters of Liberty, the United States Congress, Doctor W.B. O'Shaughnessy, Nicholas Culpepper, Doctor John Grigor, Peter Squire, Doctor J.B. Mattison, the United States Dispensatory, Doctor J.R. Reynolds, Doctor John J. Owen, Colonel Robert G. Ingersoll, Doctor W.B. Carpenter, Frances E. Willard, Robert Carter (ancestor of President Jimmy Carter), Knights of Labor, Methodist, Baptist and Catholic Churches (including Calvery Baptist Church) and 'pulpits of Churches across the country', Abraham Lincoln, Robert E. Lee, Henry Ford, Senator Lorna Milne, the American Medical Association, the Indian Hemp Drug Commission, the U.S. La Guardia Committee, the National Review, the British Government Study (1968) conducted by the Wooton Commission, the American Public Health Association, the American Bar Association, the National Council of Churches, the National Education Association, the LeDain Commission in Canada (1972), the U.S. President's Advisory Committee, the Siler Commission, Nixon's Shafer Commission, the California Academy of Family Physicians, the President's Commission on Law Enforcement and the Administration of Justice, the California Research Advisory Commission, the San Francisco Medical Society, and the United States Department of Defence.

It is also interesting to note that no similar respectable 'society' or 'legion' such as the Lincoln-Lee Legion, or the Calvery Baptist Church ever nationally organized and campaigned against people ingesting marijuana plants. This demonstrates the nonharmful nature of marijuana throughout history, unlike the many horrid harms from alcohol-drinking.

Whereas, marijuana has an international history of providing healthy medicines and foods for millions of people, alcohol has no similar favourable past, about supplying nutritional food values for human ingestion. The International Medical Congress in 1876 adopted the following conclusions concerning human ingestion of alcohol. "Alcohol is not shown to have a definate food value by any of the usual methods of chemical analysis or physiological investigation. . . . As a medicine it is not well fitted for self-prescription by the laity and the medical profession is not accountable. . . . We are of the opinion that the use of alcohol liquor as a beverage is productive of a large amount of physical disease, that it entails diseased appetites upon offspring, and that it is the cause of a large percentage of the crime and pauperism of our cities and country."[780] These are well documented scientifically substantiated conclusions.

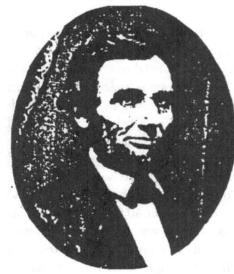

Footnote[782]

People drinking alcohol have produced many truthful harms: internal, external and to others. Democratic and morally justified man-made legislation is constitutionally intended to promote general public welfare, as identified both by the Constitution of the United States, and Abraham Lincoln's Gettysburg Address. The first official U.S. Constitution of 1789 proclaims, "We the people of the United States in order to form a more perfect union, establish justice, insure domestic tranquility . . . promote the general welfare, and secure the blessings of liberty to ourselves and our posterity do ordain and establish this Constitution."[781] Three vital principles in the previous sentence are: liberty, posterity and general welfare. Freedoms to nonharmfully add value, with no time constraints are basic constitutional rights. Hence, witholding helpful medicine from the public is a crime against humanity.

Advocating general public welfare and related freedoms to add value without harm(s) are also democratic themes of Abraham Lincoln's Gettysburg Address. On November 19, 1863 Abraham Lincoln seriously stated, "Fourscore and seven years ago our fathers brought forth on this continent a new nation conceived in liberty . . . that this nation under God shall have a new birth of freedom—and that government of the people by the people for the people shall not perish from the earth."[783] Advocating God, life, liberty, justice, humanity, freedom, posterity and 'the people' are prominent principles of popular participative democracies.

Numerous relevant reasons persist as to why public availabilities and uses of green herb marijuana plant goods should be legalized as they were for thousands of consecutive years before 1923. A primary issue is hypocricy. The very first sentence of the Canadian Charter of Right and Freedoms, "recognizes the supremacy of God" above man. God made all green herb plants, including marijuana and then directed that people use them. In Genesis or the beginning of the world, it is written, "the Lord God made the earth and the heavens . . . and every herb of the field before it grew." "AND GOD SAID BEHOLD, I have given you every herb bearing seed which is

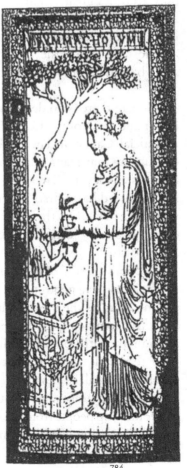

Footnote[784]

upon the face of all the earth. . . . To you it shall be for meat. . . . I have given every green herb for meat." The Encyclopedia Britannica defines marijuana as, 'an annual herb'. Also, distinctly printed on much legal currency in North America are the words, 'In God We Trust'. When we are supposed to trust in God, it is hypocritical to enforce man-made laws with any harmful punishment(s) against God's preferred green herb marijuana plants and people who nonharmfully use them.

Sections 1 and 11 of the Canadian Charter of Rights and Freedoms guarantee the right to be presumed innocent until proven guilty. It has never been proven that people using marijuana automatically or typically produce demonstrable harms. Even in 1951, official testimony before the Kefauver Committee in the United States Congress concluded, "Marijuana smokers generally . . . bother no one and have a good time. They do not stagger or fall. It has not been proved that smoking leads to crimes of violence." Also, the largest and most comprehensive marijuana study in history, the 1894 British Raj Commission Study of hashish Smokers in India concluded that marijuana use is harmless and even helpful. Several similar scientific studies all agreed including: Canada's Le Dain Commission, La Guardia, Siler, Nixon's Shafer Commission, and the California Research Advisory Commission. In a modern court of law a judge testified that marijuana is, "one of the safest therapeutically active substances known to man." With a lethal to effective dose ratio estimated at 40,000 to 1, marijuana is significantly safer than Aspirin and other pharmaceutical pills which commonly have a lethal dose only 10 times greater than their effective one. This makes marijuana thousands of times safer than Aspirin and other drug store pharmaceuticals. When speaking of marijuana smoke and hashish incenses, it is recorded, "until very recent years various aromatic substances were burned in sick rooms and hospitals where they were thought to assist oxidation and ventilation, to neutralize the effects of some bacteria and to prevent the growth of others."[785]

Where there is no demonstrable harm there should be no demonstrable punishment. This is the intent and spirit of the Canadian Charter of Rights and Freedoms. Section 1 of the Charter requires all official Canadian laws to be, 'demonstrably justified' *before* such laws are legally valid. When consuming marijuana does not produce true and proven demonstrable harms, it is *beyond* the legal limits of any law in Canada to impose harmful punishment(s) against a person when that person has not produced harm first. When no true and proven harm is first produced, laws against nonharmful user(s) are invalid, as they are beyond the legal limits of laws allowed in Canada, because they cannot be demonstrably justified, an official initial requirement of the Canadian Charter.

Sections 1 and 7 of the Canadian Charter of Rights and Freedoms guarantee the democratic right to life. Marijuana goods promote life for the people. Marijuana seeds are very biologically electron rich placing them as the most healthy and nutritious food source in the world for human consumption. Both the complete protein and the essential oils contained in marijuana seeds are, 'in ideal ratios for human nutrition'. Essential fatty acids from marijuana plants have been used to successfully treat 'terminal' cancer patients and those suffering from: kidney degeneration, immune deficiency, tuberculosis, gall stones, cardiovascular disease, glandular atrophy, dry skin and menstrual disorders. This cruel and unusual marijuana legislation demonstrably harms our democratic right promoting life, by prohibiting people from nonharmfully using beneficial marijuana foods and medicines, historically recorded as being helpful for more than 150 different medical disorders.

Harmful marijuana laws prohibiting people from using a traditionally beneficial medicine violate Section 12 of the Canadian Charter of Rights and Freedoms. "Everyone has the right not to be subjected to any cruel and unusual treatment." Witholding traditional beneficial medicine, thereby forcing people to suffer and die is unusually cruel, selfish and immoral, contrary to God's Fifth Commandment, 'Thou Shalt Not Kill'. It should be very legal for people to publicly use marijuana as a treatment with medical disorders for depression, pain or anorexia nervosa so people can be less likely to commit suicide or die from starvation or despair. In a democracy people shouldn't be legally forced to use inferior medicines having harmful side-effects and less effective results.

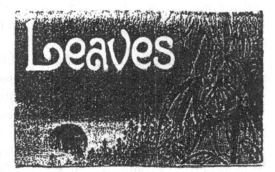

Footnote[786]

Restrictive marijuana laws also violate Section 15 of the Canadian Charter of Rights and Freedoms. Sections 1 and 15 guarantee that each Canadian, "has the right to . . . equal benefit of the law without discrimination." Obvious discrimination occurs when governmental legislation allows one relaxant alcohol, a demonstrably harm-producing relaxant, while legally prohibiting a medically helpful or health-producing relaxant (marijuana). True discrimination occurs as governmental legislation publicly allows the harmful product (alcohol) that produces more than 150 different medical harms to peoples bodies, without *even one* nutritional medical benefit, while other laws publicly prohibit more than 150 different medical benefits from ingesting marijuana plant goods. In summary, this amounts to at least 300 reasons why related harm producing laws are *not for* the people.

Also, unlike alcohol and most commercially manufactured tobacco cigarettes, smoking marijuana does not cause lung cancer. While millions of North Americans have smoked marijuana regularly, marijuana use has never produced any truthfully substantiated case of lung cancer, according to America's foremost lung expert, Dr. Donald Tashkin.

"What do the scientific facts say? Marijuana does not destroy the brain."[787] Also, smoking marijuana, "is not only pleasurable and innocuous, they claim it has certain decided health benefits. It should be legalized."[788]

Medical studies have also shown that, "marijuana does not lead to blocked airways or emphysema."[789] Similarly, an official marijuana research report published in a special two volume issue by the New England Journal of Medicine describes successful effectiveness of marijuana plant products for, "alleviating an astonishing range of physical ailments: nausea, glaucoma, autoimmune diseases like asthma and arthritis, hypertension depression, etc."[790]

Conversely, a health newsline from Ottawa (November, 1998) concludes, "Antidepressants hailed since the 1980s for having no unpleasant side-effects can cause anything from nausea to insomnia or anorexia. In a review published in the Canadian Medical Association Journal, researchers report that widely used antidepressants such as Prozac can also cause diarrhea, nervousness, anxiety and agitation. In other studies, researchers found the newer drugs called selective serotonin reuptake inhibitors are no safer or more effective than other drugs used for treating severe depression."[791] It seems logical that governments *for* the people would legally allow public uses of marijuana for treating depression and any other medical disorder. Scientific conclusions already show that public uses of marijuana for depression are safer and more effective than modern pharmaceuticals.

A marijuana research report from British Columbia in 2003 concludes, "Not only are the buds medicinal but the rest of the plant can be used. . . . Unlike alcohol and hard drugs, marijuana makes people mellow. Legalization could have positive effects. . . . Cannabis provides effective relief to those suffering from: anorexia, cancer, AIDS, stress, PMS and depression, without physical addiction."[792]

"Perhaps if more people realized what a huge industry marijuana production is already, they might be more open to a common sense solution. Marijuana is already being produced in great quantities, with none of the direct profits benefiting the taxpayers. The illegal operators make the money. The taxpayers pay for law enforcement costs."[793] Legalization would naturally benefit taxpayers, as long as no legalized intentional contamination is allowed, as with currently manufactured commercial cigarettes. Intentional contamination of food can produce cancers in peoples' bodies, contrary to democracy *for* the people.

"By not fully legalizing and regulating cannabis, the Canadian government is knowingly subsidizing organized crime to the tune of about $10 billion per year . . . wasting valuable police time and resources, wasting billions annually in taxpayers' money on enforcement, courts and corrections, witholding billions more in potential annual tax revenue, and witholding a valuable source of medicine from sick and dying Canadians."[794] This does not truthfully demonstrate a just and joyful society for the people. Witholding helpful medicine is cruel and immoral behaviour, especially in a democracy where freedom of choice to add value without harm defines liberty, a guaranteed constitutional right.

Prohibiting public medical uses of marijuana harmfully, "afflicts many Canadians, even more so our friends south of the border, nevermind that both former presidents George Washington and Thomas Jefferson grew hemp on their estates, and towns like Hempsted, N.Y. were named for it."[795]

Improving peoples' health benefits both the person and society. Healthy people have abilities to add more value, be more joyful and incur less hospitalization costs than unhealthy unhappy people. Publicly prohibiting helpful medicine contravenes constitutional rights advocating: life, liberty, happiness and security of the person. The very first sentence of Canada's Charter of Rights and Freedoms proclaims, "Canada is founded upon principles that recognize the supremacy of God." And God said, "I have given every green herb for meat . . . and thou shalt eat the herb of the field."

For humane reasons, promoting life, liberty, equality, security, joy, happiness and posterity, each person can make a difference by asking logical questions to relevant people about why we are not legally allowed to be free in our own democracy. Remember, as the friendly song says, "You Can't Be A Beacon, If Your Light Don't Shine." Each person always trying to improve things can produce a more peaceful, healthy and prosperous society, with less environmental harms from floods, winds, warming, freezing, droughts and severe weather.

Unimaginable punishments could indeed await those who do *not* support and practice God's directions. In addition to the 'Fires of Hell' there could be more horrible punishments. A

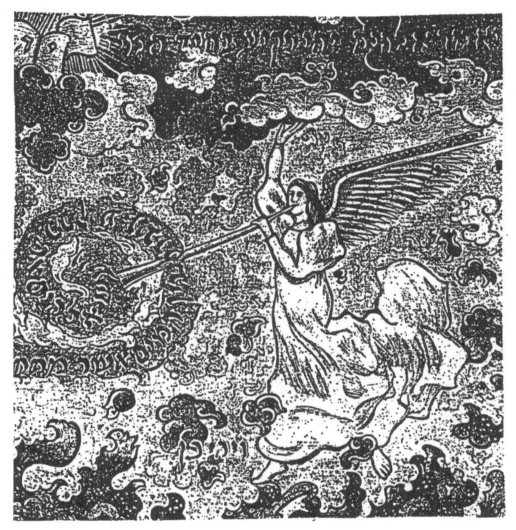

Footnote[796]

description of some horrid conditions is provided by Christ's Apostles Peter and Paul. "The Apostle Peter announcing to the public a vision said: And in another great lake full of pitch and blood and mire bubbling up, there stood men and women up to their knees. . . . The Apostle Paul relating his vision said, "And I saw another multitude of pits in the same place, and in the midst of it a river full of a multitude of men and women, and worms consumed them. But I lamented and sighing asked the angel and said: Who are these? And he said to me, "These are those who . . . did not hope in God that he was their helper." See Ante-Nicene Fathers, Vol. 9, page 160."[797] On Judgment Day, God may well ask words to the effect, "and what specifically did you do to improve the man-made legal status of my preferred green herb marijuana plants?"

BIBLIOGRAPHY

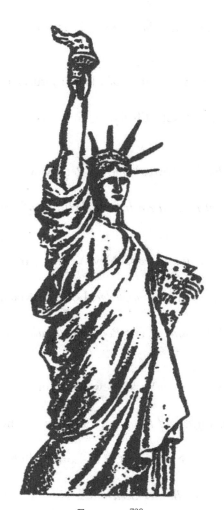

Footnote[798]

By: Joseph W. Jacob B.A., M.P.A.

ABEL, ERNEST L. *Marihuana The First Twelve Thousand Years*, New York: Plenum Press, 1980.

ACADEMIC AMERICAN ENCYCLOPEDIA. New Jersey: Arete Publishing Co., 1981.

ADAMS, JOHN. *The Founding Fathers.* New York: Harper & Row, 1961.

ALASKA HIGHWAY NEWS, Fort St. John, B.C.: Alaska Highway News, 2003.

ALLEN, EVERETT S. *The Black Ships Rumrunners of Prohibition*, Boston: Little, Brown & Co., 1979.

ALON, AZARIA. *The Natural History of the Bible*, Israel: Jerusalem Printing House, 1969.

AMERICAN SPICE TRADE ASSOCIATION. *A Treasury of Spices*, New York: American Spice Trade Association, 1956.

ANDREWS, GEORGE. *The Book of Grass*, London: Peter Owen Ltd., 1967.

ASBURY, HERBERT. *The Great Illusion An Informal History of Prohibition*, New York: Doubleday & Co., 1950.

AUGUST, E. *John Stuart Mill A Mind at Large*, New York: Charles Scribners Sons, 1935.

AYER, A.J. *The Foundations of Empirical Knowledge*, London: Macmillan & Co., 1964.

BAILEY, S. *Possession of Small Amounts of Pot Remains Illegal*, Whitehorse, Y.T.: Whitehorse Star, 2003.

BAIN, J. *Tobacco in Song and Story*, New York: New York Public Library, 1953.

BARBER, T. *LSD, Marijuana, Yoga, and Hypnosis*, Chicago: Aldine Publishing Co., 1970.

BARTH, R. *Hemp's Energy Promise*, Nelson, B.C.: Nelson Daily News, 2005.

BARTH, R. *Marc Emery and Cross-Border Seed Sales*, New Westminster, B.C.: Coquitlam Now, 2005.

BARTHELEMY, O. and MILIK, J. *Discoveries in Judean Desert I Qumran Cave*, Oxford: Clarendon Press, 1955.

BELL, M. *The Politics of Pot*, and *In Focus*, Vancouver, B.C.: Vancouver Echo, Mar. 6, 1996 and Mar. 26, 1997.

BENNETT, C., OSBURN, L. and J. *Green Gold The Tree of Life*, California: Access Unlimited, 1995.

158

BENOIT, P. *Discoveries in the Judean Desert*, Oxford: Clarendon Press, 1961.

BERRY, RALPH E. JR. and BOLAND, JAMES P. *The Economic Cost of Alcohol Abuse*, New York: Collier, 1977.

BLOOMQUIST, EDWARD R. *Marijuana The Second Trip*, Beverly Hills: Glencoe Press, 1971.

BOSWELL, R. *Edmonton Crusader Blamed For Marijuana Menace*, Edmonton, Alta.: Edmonton Journal, 2004.

BOSWELL, R. *Emily Murphy,* Calgary, Alta.: Calgary Herald, 2004.

BOSWELL, R. *How the Marijuana Menace Began*, Victoria, B.C.: Times-Colonist, 2004.

BOSWELL, R. *She Started the War on Weed*, Ottawa, Ont.: Ottawa Citizen, 2004.

BROWN, J. *Top Court to Rule on Pot Law*, Windsor, Ont.: Windsor Star, 2003.

BURNE-JONES, EDWARD. *The Beginning of the World*, London: Longmans, Green, 1902.

CANNABIS CANADA, *Marijuana is Medicine*, Vancouver, B.C.: 1996.

CARTER, MIA. *Marijuana Possession is Decriminalized in MA*, http://us-elections.suite101.com/ article.efm/small_amounts_of_marijuana_decriminalized_in_ma [2008].

CASHMAN, SEAN, D. *Prohibition The Lie of the Land*, London: Collier Macmillan, 1981.

CHAMBERS'S ENCYCLOPAEDIA A Dictionary of Universal Knowledge New Edition Volume V, London: W. & R. Chambers, 1980.

CHAMBERS'S ENCYCLOPAEDIA Volume V, London: J.B. Lippincott Co., 1924.

CHAPMAN, PAUL. *What and How It Helps*, Vancouver, B.C.: The Province, Oct. 4, 1995.

CHESHIRE, FRANK R. *The Scientific Temperance Hand-Book*, London: Lorimer & Gillies, 1891.

CLARK, NORMAN H. *The Dry Years Prohibition and Social Change*, Washington: University of Washington Press, 1988.

CLARK, R.C. *Hashish!* Los Angeles: Red Eye Press, 1998.

CLARKES, LINCOLN, *Cannabis The Truth Is On Our Side (Indica Plant)*, Vancouver, B.C.: Lincoln Clarkes, 1995.

CLARKES, LINCOLN. *Just Say Grow*, Vancouver, B.C.: Hemp B.C., 1995.

CLARKES, LINCOLN. *My Canada Includes Cannabis (Flowering Sativa Plant)*, Lincoln Clarkes, 1994.

CONNEL P.H. and DORN N. *Cannabis and Man Psychological and Clynical Aspects and Patterns of Use*, New York: Churchill Livingstone, 1975.

CONRAD, CHRIS. *Hemp Lifeline to the Future*, California: Creative Xpressions Publications, 1994.

CONRAD, LAWRENCE I. *The Western Medical Tradition*, New York: Cambridge University Press, 1995.

COOPER, MARTY. (Sung By: Fargo, Donna) *You Can't Be A Beacon If Your Light Don't Shine*, Willowdale, Ont., MCA Records, 1977.

CORBETT, J.E. *Turned On By God*, Richmond, Virginia: John Knox Press, 1971.

CUMMINS, JOHN. *The Voyage of Christopher Columbus,* New York: St. Martin's Press, 1980.

DAICHES, DAVID. *Moses Man In the Wilderness*, London: Weidenfeld and Nicolson, 1975.

DANIELS, W.H. *The Temperance Reform And Its Great Reformers*, New York: Nelson & Phillips, 1878.

DARE, MICHAEL (Billboard Magazine). *The 90's The Hemp Video*, Boulder, Colorado: 1990.

DICKENS, CEDRIC. *Drinking With Dickens*, England: Mears, Caldwell, Hacker Ltd., 1980.

DREHER, MELANIE C. *Working Men and Ganja, Marijuana Use in Rural Jamaica*, Philadelphia: *Institute For the Study of Human Issues*, 1982.

DREY, RUDOLF E. *Apothecary Jars*, London: Faber & Faber, 1978.

DUNLOP, RICHARD. *Doctors of the American Frontier*, New York: Doubleday & Co., 1965.

ENCYCLOPAEDIA BRITANNICA VOLUME 11, Chicago: William Benton Publisher, 1972.

ENCYCLOPAEDIA BRITANNICA VOLUME 18, Chicago, William Benton Publishers, 1972.

ERICKSON, PATRICIA G. *Cannabis Criminals The Social Effects of Punishment on Drug Users,* Toronto: T.H. Best Printing Co., 1980.

EVEREST, ALLAN S. *Rum Across the Border*, New York: Syracuse University Press, 1978.

EVERYMAN'S ENCYCLOPAEDIA VOLUME 6, London: J.M. Dent & Sons, 1967.

FAIRHOLT, F.W. *Tobacco Its History and Associations*, London: Chapman & Hall, 1859.

FINE, RALPH ADAM. *Mary Jane Versus Pennsylvania*, New York: The McCall Publishing Co., 1970.

FINLEY, DAVID EDWARD. *A Standard of Excellence*, Washington, D.C.: Smithsonian Institution Press, 1973.

FISCHER-RIZZI, S. *The Complete Incense Book*, New York: Sterling Publishing Co. Inc., 1998.

FLOWERS, TOM. *Marijuana Herbal Cookbook*, Berkeley, California: Flowers Publishing, 1995.

FORD, THOMAS K. *The Apothecary in Eighteenth Century Williamsburg*, Williamsburg Publications, 1965.

FREDEMAN, P. *Pre-Raphaelitism,* Cambridge, Massachusetts: Harvard University Press, 1965.

FREUND, JOHN E. and WILLIAMS, FRANK J. *Freund and Williams' Modern Business Statistics,* New Jersey: Penntice-Hall, Inc., 1969.

GARROD, STAN. *Samuel De Champlain*, Don Mills, Ontario: Fitzhenry & Whiteside, 1981. Cover.

GELLER, ALLEN and BOAS, MAXWELL. *The Drug Beat*, New York: Cowles Book Co., 1969.

GOLDMAN, ALBERT. *Grass Roots Marijuana in America Today*, New York: Harper & Row, 1979.

GORDON, SEAN. *Marijuana, the Debate*, Montreal Que.: The Gazette, 2002.

GORMAN, PETER. (High Times) *Marijuana and AIDS*, New York: Trans-High Co., 1994.

GOUGH, JOHN B. *Platform Echoes: Living Truths For Head and Heart*, Hartford: A.D. Worthington & Co., 1886.

GOVERNMENT OF CANADA. *Canadian Charter or Rights and Freedoms*, Ottawa: Publications Canada, 1982.

GOVERNMENT OF CANADA. *The Charter or Rights and Freedoms*, Ottawa: Publications Canada, 1982.

GRINSPOON, LESTER (M.D.) *Marijuana Reconsidered*, Massachusetts: Harvard University Press, 1971.

HALSEY, W.D. *Collier's Encyclopedia Volume 9*, U.S.A.: P.F. Collier, 1972.

HARVEY, W.H. *The Book*, Rogers, Arkansas: The Mundus Publishing Co., 1930.

HEMP MAGAZINE The Environmental Newspaper, Houston, Texas: Feb. and March, 1997.

HEMPEL, CARL G. *Philosophy of Natural Science*, New Jersey: Prentice-Hall, 1966.

HERER, JACK. *Hemp and the Marihuana Conspiracy*, California: Queen of Clubs Publishing, 1993.

HIGH TIMES, New York: Trans-High Co., Feb. & Nov. 1996, and Apr. and May, 1997.

HIMMELSTEIN, J. *The Strange Career of Marijuana*, Connecticut: Greenwood Press, 1983.

HUNTER, R. *The Imperial Encyclopaedic Dictionary*, London: Dictionary and Cyclopedia Co., 1901.

INTERNATIONAL BIBLE SOCIETY. *The Holy Bible*, Michigan: Zondervan Bible Publishers, 1988.

JACOBI, JOLANDE. *Paracelsus Selected Writings*, London: Routledge & Kegan Ltd., 1951.

KANE, HARNETT T. *Plantation Parade*, New York: William Morrow and Co., 1945.

KEEN, BENJAMIN. *The Life of the Admiral Christopher Columbus*, New Jersey: Rutgers University Press, 1959.

LARSEN, DANA. *Bill C-8: The Controlled Drugs and Substances Act*, Vancouver, B.C.: Cannabis Canada, May, 1996.

LAUNERT, EDMUND. *Perfume and Pomanders*, Europe: Potterton Books, 1987.

LAVERGNE, ALYCIA and ROBINSON, AMANDA. *Mellow Out on Pot Laws*, Chilliwack, B.C.: Chilliwack Times, 2003.

LOCKE, GEORGE H. *The World Book*, Toronto: W.F. Quarrie & Co., 1923.

LOURIA, DONALD B. (M.D.) *The Drug Scene*, New York: McGraw Hill Book Co., 1968.

MARSTON, SIR CHARLES. *The Bible Is True*, London: Eyre and Spottiswoode, 1934.

MAYER, CAROLINE. *DEA Puts the Bite on Hemp Chips*, Montreal, Que.: The Gazette, 2002.

MAZLISH, BRUCE. *James and John Stuart Mill*, New York: Basic Books Inc., 1975.

MERLIN, MARK D. *Man and Marijuana Some Aspects of Their Ancient Relationship*, New Jersey: Fairleigh Dickinson University Press, 1972.

MICROSOFT INTERNET EXPLORER. *The Complete History of Cannabis in Canada*, Microsoft Internet Explorer, Winnipeg: 1996.

MIDDLETON, GREG. *Quit Filing Drug-Possession Charges, Vancouver Cops Told Users Off the Hook*, Vancouver, B.C.: The Province, 1995.

MILLER, CAROL and WIRTSHAFTER, DON. *The Hemp Seed Cookbook*, Ohio: The Ohio Hempery Inc., 1994.

MONTREAL MUSEUM OF FINE ATRS, *Boites a Encens Japonaises Redecouvertes*, Montreal: The Georges Clemenceau Kogo Collection, 1978.

MONTREAL MUSEUM OF FINE ARTS, *Exhibition of Kogo*, Montreal: Montreal Museum of Fine Arts, 1978.

MOORE, CHARLES. *Pot Should Be Legal*, Halifax, N.S.: Daily News, 2002.

MORRISON, JAMES H. *Tempered By Rum*, Porters Lake, Nova Scotia: Pottersfield Press, 1988.

MOSBY INC. *Mosby's Medical, Nursing & Allied Health Dictionary* (Sixth Edition), Missouri: 2002.

NANAIMO DAILY NEWS. *Legalized Marijuana Would Help*, Nanaimo, B.C.: Nanaimo Daily News, 2001.

NEW STANDARD ENCYCLOPEDIA Volume 4, Chicago: Standard Educational Co., 1995.

OTTAWA CITIZEN, Ottawa, Ont.: Ottawa Citizen, 2000.

PEARSON, C. *Activist Says Pot Sales Were Legal*, Windsor, Ont.: Windsor Star, 2004.

PEAT, MARWICK, MITCHELL & CO. *Marijuana A Study of State Policies and Penalties*, Washington, D.C.: U.S. Department of Justice, 1977.

POWELL, B. and COCKBURN, N. *Prosecutors Uncertain How They Will React*, Toronto, Ont.: Toronto Star, 2003.

RAISON, ARNOLD V. *Brief History of Pharmacy in Canada*, Canadian Pharmaceutical Journal, 1967.

RANDALL, J.G. *Lincoln The President*, New York: Dodd, Mead & Co., 1956.

By: Joseph W. Jacob B.A., M.P.A.

RATHBURN, MARY. *Brownie Mary's Marijuana Cookbook*, San Francisco: Trail of Smoke Publishing, 1993.

RHODEHAMEL, JOHN H. *Foundations of Freedom*, Los Angeles: Constitutional Rights Foundation, 1991.

RICHMOND, A.B. *Intemperance and Crime Leaves From the Diary of an Old Lawyer,* Cleveland: J.B. Savage, 1883.

ROBINSON, ROWAN. *The Great Book of Hemp*, Rochester, Vermont: Park Street Press, 1996.

ROMI, ADAM. *Marijuana Law Ignores Benefits*, Regina, Sask.: Leader Post, 2003.

ROSENTHAL, ED. *Marijuana Growing Tips*, San Francisco: Quick American Publishing, 1975.

ROTH, JUNE. *Old-Fashioned Candymaking*, Chicago: Henry Regnery Co., 1974.

ROULAC, JOHN W. *Industrial Hemp*, Ojai, California: Hemptech, 1995.

ROUSE JR. PARKE. *Pioneers Life in Colonial Virginia*, New York: Hastings House Publishers, 1968.

RUBIN, VERA. *Cannabis and Culture*, Paris: Mouton Publishers, 1975.

SCHACHNER, NATHAN. *Thomas Jefferson*, London: Thomas Yoseloff Inc., 1957.

SCHWARCZ, JOE. *Despite Decades of Propaganda, Cannabis is Proving its Worth*, Montreal, Que.: The Gazette, 2000.

SENATE OF CANADA. *Public Hearings For Bill C-8, Transcripts*, Ottawa: 1996.

SHERMAN, C. and SMITH, A. *Highlights An Illustrated History of Cannabis*, Toronto: Ten Speed Press, 1999.

SHERMAN, ORI. *The Creation*, New York: Dial Books, 1990.

SILVERBERG, ROBERT. *The Dawn of Medicine*, New York: G.P. Putnam's Sons, 1966.

SIMKINS, FRANCIS B. *A History of the South*, New York: Alfred A. Knopf, 1956.

SIRAISI, NANCY G. *Medieval and Early Rennaissance Medicine*, London: University of Chicago, 1990.

SLOMAN, LARRY. *The History of Marihuana in America Reefer Madness*, New York: Bobbs-Merrill Co., 1979.

SMITH, MICHAEL. *The Afternoon Tea Book*, New York: 1986.

STAMM, J.J. and ANDREW, M.E. *The Ten Commandments in Recent Research*, London: SCM Press, 1962.

STEVEACRE, F.W. *Tea and Tea Drinking*, London: Sir Isaac Pitman and Sons, 1929.

STRATTON, DEBORAH. *Candlesticks*, London: Pitman, 1976.

STREET-PORTER, JANET and TIM. *The British Teapot*, London: Angus & Robertson Publishers, 1981.

SUDBURY STAR, *The Alarming Global Reach of U.S. Law*, Sudbury Ont.: Sudbury Star, 2005.

THE BOOK OF KNOWLEDGE, New York: Grolier, 1969.

THE CALGARY HERALD, Calgary, Alta.: Calgary Herald, 1996, 1998, and 2004.

THE CENTURY DICTIONARY AND CYCLOPEDIA, New York: The Century Co., 1904.

THE ENCYCLOPEDIA AMERICANA INTERNATIONAL EDITION, Volume 22, Connecticut: Grolier, 1982.

THE ENCYCLOPEDIA BRITANNICA A Dictionary of Arts, Sciences, and General Literature Ninth Edition, Volume XI, Edinburgh: Adam & Charles Black, 1880.

THE MORAL EVOLUTION ISSUE POT SHOT #15, Vancouver, B.C.: Hemp B.C. 1998.

THE NEW EDUCATOR ENCYCLOPEDIA VOLUMES 3 & 5, Toronto: General Press, 1956.

THE NEW INTERNATIONAL ENCYCLOPAEDIA VOLUME XI, New York: Dodd Mead & Co., 1922.

THE NEW WEBSTER ENCYCLOPEDIC DICTIONARY OF THE ENGLISH LANGUAGE, Chicago: Consolidated Book Publishers, 1971.

THE OXFORD ENGLISH DICTIONARY VOLUME VII, Oxford, England: The Clarendon Press, 1933.

THE PROVINCE, Vancouver, B.C.: Pacific Press, 1996, 1997, and 1998.

THE ROYAL COLLEGE OF PHYSICIANS *A Great and Growing Evil*, London: Tavistock, 1987.

THE RUSHLIGHT CLUB. *Early Lighting*, Connecticut: Finlay Bros. Inc., 1972.

By: Joseph W. Jacob B.A., M.P.A.

THE SECRETARY, DEPARTMENT OF HEALTH, EDUCATION, AND WELFARE, AND SUBCOMMITTEE ON ALCOHOLISM AND NARCOTICS OF THE COMMITTEE ON LABOR AND PUBLIC WELFARE, UNITED STATES SENATE. *Marihuana and Health A Report to the Congress*, Washington, D.C.: U.S. Government Printing Office, 1971.

THE TORONTO STAR, Toronto, Ont.: Toronto Star, 1996, 1997, 1998, and 2003.

THE VANCOUVER SUN, Vancouver, B.C.: Pacific Press, 1995, 1998, and 2000.

THE WORLD BOOK ENCYCLOPEDIA. VOLUME 5 (D), London: World Book Inc., 1994.

TROTTER, THOMAS (L.D.S.) *Life Pictures From Rum's Gallery*, Toronto: William Briggs, 1886.

TROWBRIDGE, J.T. *The South*, Connecticut: L. Stebbins, 1867.

TUCKER FETTNER, ANN. *Potpourri Incense*, New York: Workman Publishing Co., 1977.

VACHON, ANDRE, *Records of Our History*, Ottawa: Canadian Government Publishing Centre, 1985.

VEITH, ILZA. *Huang Ti Nei Ching Su Wen*, Los Angeles: University of California Press, 1996.

WEATHERALL, M. *In Search of a Cure*, New York: Oxford University Press, 1990.

WHITFIELD J. and BELL J. *The Colonial Physician*, New York: Science History Publications, 1975.

WILLARD, FRANCES E. *How I Learned to Ride the Bicycle*, Sunnyvale, California: Fair Oaks Publishing, 1991.

WILSON, JAMES GRANT. *Appletons' Cyclopaedia of American Biography*, New York: D. Appleton & Co., 1989.

WINSTON, RICHARD and CLARA. *Science and Secrets of Early Medicine*, London: Thames and Hudson, 1962.

WOOD, DANIEL. *War Without Winners Cops and Addicts Agree That the War on Drugs is Fatally Flawed*, Vancouver, B.C.: Georgia Straight, 1995.

WOODHAM-SMITH, CECIL. *Queen Victoria*, Great Britain: Hamish Hamilton Ltd., 1972.

WOODROW, MARTIN. *People From the Bible*, Connecticut: Morehouse-Barlow, 1987.

WORLD BOOK ENCYCLOPEDIA VOLUME 11 (J-K), Chicago: World Book Inc., 1995.

WORLD BOOK ENCYCLOPEDIA VOLUME 19 (T), Chicago: World Book Inc., 2007.

WORLD HEALTH ORGANIZATION. *The Use of Cannabis Report of a WHO Scientific Group Technical Report Series NO. 478*, Geneva: 1971.

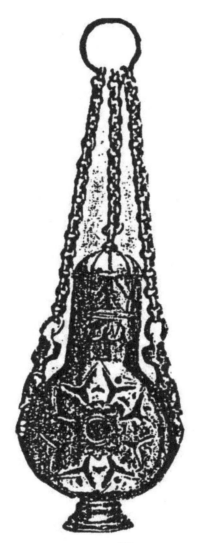

Footnote[799]

The Public Incense Altar on the Front
Cover is Typical of Rock or Stone Altars
Used For Thousands of Years in Olden Days
For Respectfully Burning Marijuana Resins
(Hashes), Buds, Leaves and Flowers, Making
Holy Smoke For All Free-Choice Participants

INDEX

A

D

175

E

F

H

M

S

ALCOHOL

It's Not the Cane in Rum, It's Not the Grain in Rye
It's Not The Fruit in Wine, It's Not the Hops in Beer
But There's One Thing Clear, It's the Alcohol That Kills

Drinking Alcohol is Harmful, Deceiving as Can Be
Destroying Lives and Taking Fun from Folks Like You and Me
Now Alcohol's So Sneeky as it Eats Alone
Killing Nerves and Organs Right Down to the Bone

It's Not the Cane in Rum, It's Not the Grain in Rye
It's Not the Fruit in Wine, It's Not the Hops in Beer
But There's One Thing Clear, It's the Alcohol That Kills

Alcohol Destroys Continuously, It Doesn't Help Things Grow
It Makes the Mind Go Foggy and Makes the Body Slow
But Then It's Power Time and the Mouth Gets Mean
And Soon a Friend is Gone
And Alcohol, It's Harms and Hurts Are There Causing the Fall

It's Not the Cane in Rum, It's Not the Grain in Rye
It's Not the Fruit in Wine, It's Not the Hops in Beer
But There's One Thing Clear, It's the Alcohol That Kills

Now if We Like Our Organs, Our Kidneys Hearts and Eyes
Then Stay Away From Alcohol and We'll Be Happily Surprised
First We Get Our Health Back, Then We Get Good Friends
Then We Make Decisions That Make a Lot of Sense

It's Not the Cane in Rum, It's Not the Grain in Rye
It's Not the Fruit in Wine, It's Not the Hops in Beer
But There's One Thing Clear, It's the Alcohol That Kills
Continuously . . .

MARIJUANA

Marijuana Plants are Great Indeed, Put on Earth For Everyone
Some Folks Like Em For Relaxation, Others Use Em to Get Things Done

Marijuana Helps a Person Concentrate to Do a Better Job
It Reduces Stress, It Reduces Pains
It Tends to Make Us Get Along

Marijuana Use Improves Appetites and Reduces Migraine Headaches
It's Also Good For Coughs and Colds
And For Taking Pains From Earaches

Marijuana Use Reduces High Blood Pressure
And Is Also Great For Depression, It Makes a Person Calm
It Makes a Person Think and It's Even Good for Vision

Marijuana Helps With Rheumatism and Asthma and Arthritis
Marijuana Makes a Person More Humane
And Many Say They Just Plain Like It

Marijuana's Good, Marijuana's Fine
It's the Laws That Are a Problem
Marijuana Laws Cause Demonstrable Harms
As They Violate Our Democratic Rights and Freedoms

The Canadian Charter of Rights and Freedoms
Guarantees the Right to Liberty
When No Harm is Done and We're Having Fun
Well That's Democratic Liberty

So Let's All Have a Great Ole Time, Just Trying to Improve Things
Let's Avoid Contradictions and Hypocrises
Always Being Truthful and Persistent

Marijuana Plants Are Great Indeed, Put on Earth For Everyone
Some Folks Like Em For Relaxation, Others Use Em to Get Things Done
So Let's Keep On Gettin' Nice Things Done. Ya!

FOOTNOTES

Footnote[800]

1   Burne-Jones, E. *The Beginning of the World*, London: Longmans, Green & Co., 1902. pp. 5-19.

2   Woodrow, M. *People From the Bible*, Connecticut: Morehouse-Barlow, 1897. p.1.

3   Burne-Jones, E. *The Beginning of the World*, London: Longmans, Green & Co., 1902. pp. 5-19.

4   Clarkes, L. *Cannabis The Truth Is On Our Side*, (*Indica Plant*), Vanc.: L. Clarkes, 1995. Cover.

5   Clarkes, L. *My Canada Includes Cannabis* (*Flowering Sativa Plant*) Lincoln Clarkes, 1994. Cover.

6   *The Encyclopaedia Britannica Volume XI*, Edinburgh: 1880. p. 647.

7   Burne-Jones, E. *The Beginning of the World*, London: Longmans, Green & Co., 1902. p. 19.

8   Ibid. p. 12.

9   Ibid. p. 9.

10 Ibid. p. 12.

11 Ibid. p. 8.

12 Rubin, V. *Cannabis and Culture*, Paris: Mouton Publishers, 1975. p. 44.

13 Abel, E. *Marihuana The First Twelve Thousand Years*, New York: Plenum Press, 1980. p. 4.

14 Ibid. p. 4.

15 Barthelemy, O. *Discoveries in the Judean Desert I Qumran Cave*, Oxford: Clarendon, 1955. p. 31.

16 Abel, E. *Marihuana The First Twelve Thousand Years*, New York: Plenum Press, 1980. p. 5.

17 Daiches, D. *Moses Man in the Wilderness*, London: Weidenfeld and Nicolson, 1975. p. 17.

18 Rubin, V. *Cannabis and Culture*, Paris: Mouton Publishers, 1975. p. 52.

19 Ibid. p. 55.

20 Ibid. p. 55.

21 Goldman, A. *Grass Roots Marijuana in America Today*, New York: Harper & Row, 1979. p. 35.

22 Ibid. p. 35.

23 Rubin, V. *Cannabis and Culture*, Paris: Mouton Publishers, 1975. p. 53.

24 Woodrow, M. *People From the Bible*, Connecticut: Morehouse-Barlow, 1987. p. 134.

25 Rubin, V. *Cannabis and Culture*, Paris: Mouton Publishers, 1975, p. 53.

26 Ibid. p. 53.

27 Abel, E. *Marihuana The First Twelve Thousand Years*, New York: Plenum Press, 1980. p. 10.

28 Ibid. p. 10.

29 Ibid. p. 12.

30 Veith, I. *Huang Ti Nei Ching Su Wen*, Los Angeles: University of California, 1966. p. 1.

31 Abel, E. *Marihuana The First Twelve Thousand Years*, New York: Plenum Press, 1980, p. 12.

32 United States Senate. *Marihuana and Health A Report to the Congress*, Washington, D.C.: U.S. Government Printing Office, 1971. p. 53.

33 Silverberg, R. *The Dawn of Medicine*, New York: G.P. Putnam, 1966. p. 117.

34 United States Senate. *Marihuana and Health A Report to the Congress*, Washington, D.C.: U.S. Government Printing Office, 1971. p. 53.

35 Abel, E. *Marihuana The First Twelve Thousand Years*, New York: Plenum Press, 1980. p. 18.

36 Herer, J. *Hemp & The Marihuana Conspiracy*, Van Nuys: Queen of Clubs 1993. p. 53.

37 Abel, E. *Marihuana The First Twelve Thousand Years*, New York: Plenum Press, 1980. p. 15.

38 Herer, J. *Hemp & The Marihuana Conspiracy*, Van Nuys: Queen of Clubs, 1993. p. 53.

39 Rubin, V. *Cannabis and Culture*, Paris: Mouton Publishers, 1975. p. 40.

40 Tucker Fettner, A. *Potpourri, Incense*, New York: Workman Publishing, 1977. p. 104.

41 Rubin, V. *Cannabis and Culture*, Paris: Mouton Publishers, 1975. p. 40.

42 Ibid. p. 44.

43 Bennett, C., Osburn, L. & J. *Green Gold The Tree of Life*, California: Access Unlimited, 1995. p. 95.

44 Tucker Fettner, A, *Potpourri, Incense*, New York: Workman Publishing, 1977. p. 104.

45 Rubin, V. *Cannabis and Culture*, Paris: Mouton Publishers, 1975. p. 44.

46 Montreal Museum of Fine Arts, *Exhibition of Kogo*, Montreal: 1978. p. 59.

47 Stamm, J. and Andrew, M. *The Ten Commandments in Recent Research*, London: SCM, 1962. p. 5.

48 Burne-Jones, E. *The Beginning Of The World*, London: Longmans, Green & Co., 1902, p. 19.

49 Rubin, V. *Cannabis and Culture*, Paris: Mouton Publishers, 1977. p. 44.

50 International Bible Society. *The Holy Bible*, Grand Rapids: Zondervan, 1988. p. 832.

51 Rubin, V. *Cannabis and Culture*, Paris: Mouton Publishers, 1975. p. 41.

52 Silverberg, R. *The Dawn of Medicine*, New York: G.P. Putnams Sons, 1966. Cover.

53 Bennett, C. and Osburn, L.&J. *Green Gold The Tree of Life*, Cal., Access Unlimited, 1995. p. 109.

54 Ibid. pp. 109-110.

55 Rubin, V. *Cannabis and Culture*, Paris: Mouton Publishers, 1975. p. 114.

56 Launert, E. *Perfumes and Pomanders*, Europe: Potterton, 1987. p. 11.

57 Rubin, V. *Cannabis and Culture*, Paris: Mouton Publishers, 1975. pp. 44-45.

58 Ibid. p. 40.

59 Daiches, D. *Moses Man in the Wilderness*, London: Weidenfeld & Nicolson, 1975. p. 249.

60 Rubin, V. *Cannabis and Culture*, Paris: Mouton Publishers, 1975. p. 42.

61 Ibid. p. 42.

62 Ibid. p. 2.

63 *The Encyclopedia Britannica Volume XI*, Edinburgh: 1880. p. 647.

64 Launert, E. *Perfumes and Pomanders*, Europe: Potterton, 1987. p. 12.

65 Rubin, V. *Cannabis and Culture*, Paris: Mouton Publishers, 1975. p. 2.

66 Ibid. p. 42.

67 Abel, E. *Marihuana The First Twelve Thousand Years*, New York: Plenum Press, 1980. p. 19.

68 Rubin, V. *Cannabis and Culture*, Paris: Mouton Publishers, 1975. p. 45.

69 Winston, R. & C. *Science and Secrets of Early Medicine*, London: Thames & Hudson, 1962. p. 242.

70 Bennett, C., Osburn, L. & J. *Green Gold The Tree of Life*, California: Access Unlimited, 1995. p. 55.

71 Rubin, V. *Cannabis and Culture*, Paris: Mouton Publishers, 1975. p. 45.

72 Abel, E. *Marihuana The First Twelve Thousand Years*, New York: Plenum Press, 1980. pp. 4-5.

73 Ibid. p. 5.

74 Ibid. p. 5.

75 Ibid. p. 4.

76 Bennett, C. Osburn, L.&J. *Green Gold The Tree of Life*, Cal: Access Unlimited 1995. pp. 21-22.

77 Tucker Fettner, A. *Potpourri, Incense*, New York: Workman Publishing, 1977. p. 111.

78 Bennett C, and Osburn L.&J. *The Tree of Life*, Cal: Access Unlimited, 1995. p. 143.

79 Bloomquist, E. *Marijuana The Second Trip*, Beverly Hills: Glencoe Press, 1971. pp. 18-19.

80 Abel, E. *Marihuana The First Twelve Thousand Years*, New York: Plenum, 1980. p. 61.

81 Launert, E. *Perfume and Pomanders*, Europe: Potterton, 1987. p. 150.

82 Abel, E. *Marihuana The First Twelve Thousand Years*, New York: Plenum, 1980. p. 31.

83 Ibid. p. 97.

84 Ibid. p. 97.

85 August, E. *John Stuart Mill A Mind At Large*, New York: Charles Schribner, 1935. p. 31.

86 Rosenthal, E. *Marihuana Growing Tips*, San Fran: Quick American Publishing, 1986. p. 69.

87 Grinspoon, L. *Marihuana Reconsidered*, Cambridge: Harvard Univ. Press, 1971. p. 220.

88 Bennett, C., Osburn, L. & J. *Green Gold The Tree of Life*, California: Access Unlimited, 1995. p. 19.

89 Launert, E. *Perfume and Pomanders*, Europe: Potterton, 1987. p. 17.

90 Bennett, C., Osborne, L. & J. *Green Gold The Tree of Life*, California: Access Unlimited, 1995. p. 386.

91 Ibid. p. 387.

92 Ibid. p. 387.

93 Ibid. pp. 387 and 394.

94 Meyer, C. *Sachets, Potpourri & Incense*, Illinois: Meyerbooks, 1986. p. 3.

95 Bennett, C., Osburn, L.&J. *Green Gold The Tree of Life*, Cal: Access Unlimited, 1995. p. 396.

96 Ibid. pp. 396-397.

97 Ibid. p. 387.

98 Edersheim, A. *Jesus The Messiah*, London: 1890. Insert.

99 Bennett, C., Osburn, L. & J. *Green Gold The Tree of Life*, California: Access Unlimited, 1995. p. 177.

100 Bennett, C., Osburn, L.&J. *Green Gold The Tree of Life*, Cal: Access Unlimited, 1995. p. 389.

101 Ibid. p. 400.

102 Andrews, G. *The Book of Grass*, London: Peter Owen, 1967. p. 1.

103 Bennett, C., Osburn, L.&J. *Green Gold The Tree of Life*, Cal: Access Unlimited, 1995. pp. 401-402.

104 Conrad, L. *The Western Medical Tradition*, New York: Cambridge University, 1995. p. 59.

105 Bloomquist, E. *Marijuana The Second Grip*, Beverly Hills: Glencoe Press, 1971. pp. 19-20.

106 Ibid. p. 20.

[107] Geller, A. & Boas, M. *The Drug Beat*, New York: Cowles Book Co., 1969. p. 82.

[108] Abel, E. *Marihuana The First Twelve Thousand Years*, New York: Plenum, 1980. p. 12.

[109] Ibid. p. 12.

[110] Bennett, C., Osburn, L. & J. *Green Gold The Tree of Life*, California: Access Unlimited, 1995. p. 119.

[111] Ibid. p. 121.

[112] Abel, E. *Marihuana The First Twelve Thousand Years*, New York: Plenum, 1980, p. 61.

[113] Ibid. p. 54.

[114] Ibid. p. 61.

[115] Street-Porter, J. & T. *The British Teapot*, London: Angus and Robertson, 1981. p. 16.

[116] Abel, E. *Marihuana The First Twelve Thousand Years*, New York: Plenum, 1980. p. 20.

[117] Street-Porter, J. & T. *The British Teapot*, London: Angus and Robertson, 1981. p. 116.

[118] Rubin, V. *Cannabis and Culture*, Paris: Mouton Publishers, 1975. p. 56.

[119] Bloomquist, E. *Marijuana The Second Trip*, Beverly Hills: Glencoe Press, 1971. p. 20.

[120] Bennett, C., Osburn, L. & J. *Green Gold The Tree Of Life*, California: Access Unlimited, 1995. p. 268.

[121] Benoit, P. *Discoveries in the Judean Desert*, Oxford: Clarendon Press, 1961. p. 6.

[122] Bennett, C., Osburn. L. & J. *Green Gold The Tree of Life*, Cal.: Access Unlimited: 1995. pp. 268-269.

[123] Fairholt, F.W. *Tobacco Its History and Associations*, London: Chapman, 1859. p. 41.

[124] Bennett, C., Osburn, L. & J. *Green Gold The Tree of Life*, Cal.: Access Unlimited, 1995. pp. 227-228.

[125] Abel E. *Marihuana The First Twelve Thousand Years*, New York: Plenum, 1980. p. 19.

[126] Ibid. p. 19.

[127] Ibid. p. 19.

[128] Merlin, M.D. *Man and Marihuana*, New Jersey: Fairleigh Dickinson University, 1972. p. 49.

[129] Jacobi, J. *Paracelsus Selected Writings*, London: Routledge & Kegan Ltd., 1951. p. 164.

[130] Merlin, M.D. *Man and Marihuana*, New Jersey, Fairleigh Dickenson University 1972. p. 49.

[131] Siraisi, N. *Medieval & Early Rennaissance Medicine*, London: University of Chicago Press, 1990. p. 144.

[132] Bennett, C., Osburn, L. & J. *Green Gold The Tree of Life*, Cal: Access Unlimited, 1995. p. 195.

[133] Ibid. p. 221.

[134] Alon, A. *The Natural History of the Bible*, Isreal: Jerusalem Printing House, 1969. p. 23.

[135] Abel, E. *Marijuana The First Twelve Thousand Years*, New York: Plenam, 1980. p. 97.

[136] Ibid. p. 97.

[137] Ibid. p. 97.

[138] Ibid. p. 97.

[139] Launert, E. *Perfume and Pomanders*, Europe: Potterton, 1987. p. 12.

[140] Herer, J. *Hemp & The Marihuana Conspiracy*, Van Nuys: Queen of Clubs, 1993. p. 55.

[141] Ibid. p. 55.

[142] Herer, J. *Hemp & The Marihuana Conspiracy*, Van Nuys: Queen of Clubs, 1993. p. 9.

[143] Ibid. p. 42.

[144] Ibid. p. 42.

[145] Ibid. p. 42.

[146] Keen, B. *The Life of the Admiral Christopher Columbus*, New Jersey: Rutgers Univ., 1959. p. 79.

[147] Rosenthal, E. *Marijuana Growing Tips*, San Francisco: Quick American Publishing, 1986. p. 65.

[148] Cummins, J. *The Voyage of Christopher Columbus*, New York: St. Martin's Press, 1992. p. 89.

[149] Abel, E. *Marihuana The First Twelve Thousand Years*, New York: Plenum, 1980. p. 19.

[150] Ibid. p. 20.

[151] Ibid. p. 20.

[152] Ibid. p. 21.

[153] Ibid. p. 21.

[154] Ibid. p. 21.

[155] Montreal Museum of Fine Arts. *Exhibition of Kogo*, Montreal: 1978. p. 21.

[156] Abel, E. *Marihuana The First Twelve Thousand Years*, New York: Plenum, 1980. p. 21.

[157] Rubin, V. *Cannabis and Culture*, Paris: Mouton Publishers, 1975. p. 46.

[158] Abel, E. *Marihuana The First Twelve Thousand Years*, New York: Plenum, 1980. pp. 72-73.

[159] Ibid. p. 73.

[160] *Collier's Encyclopedia Volume 9*, USA: P.F. Collier & Son, 1972. p. 95.

[161] Abel, E. *Marihuana The First Twelve Thousand Years*, New York: Plenum, 1980. p. 73.

[162] Grinspoon, L. *Marijuana Reconsidered*, Cambridge, Mass: Harvard University Press, 1971. p. 11.

[163] Jacobi, J. *Paracelsus, Selected Writings*, London: Routledge & Kegan, 1951. p. 190.

[164] Abel, E. *Marihuana The First Twelve Thousand Years*, New York: Plenum, 1980. p. 97.

[165] Garrod, S. *Samuel de Champlain*, Don Mills, Ont.: Fitzhenry & Whiteside, 1981. Cover.

[166] Abel, E. *Marihuana The First Twelve Thousand Years*, New York: Plenum, 1980. p. 97.

[167] Ibid. p. 97.

[168] Raison, A. *Brief History of Pharmacy in Canada*, Canadian Pharmaceutical Journal, 1967. p. 25.

[169] Ibid. p. 25.

[170] Andrews, G. *The Book of Grass*, London: Peter Owen Ltd., 1967. p. 115.

[171] Abel, E. *Marihuana The First Twelve Thousand Years*, New York: Plenum, 1980. p. 98.

[172] Vachon, A. *Records of Our History*, Ottawa: Canadian Government Publishing Centre, 1985. p. 44.

[173] Abel, E. *Marihuana The First Twelve Thousand Years*, New York: Plenum, 1980. p. 98.

[174] Ibid. p. 98.

[175] Ibid. p. 98.

[176] Ibid. p. 99.

[177] Ibid. p. 99.

[178] Fairholt, F.W. *Tobacco Its History and Associations*, London: Chapman, 1859. p. 95.

[179] Rubin, V. *Cannabis and Culture*, Paris: Mouton Publishers, 1975. pp. 45-46.

[180] Grinspoon, L. *Marihuana Reconsidered*, Cambridge, Massachusetts: Harvard University, 1971. p. 11.

[181] Ibid. p. 11.

[182] Ibid. p. 11.

[183] Abel, E. *Marihuana The First Twelve Thousand Years*, New York: Plenum, 1980. p. 78.

[184] Ibid. p. 78.

[185] Ibid. p. 78.

186 Ibid. p. 79.
187 Whitfield, J. *The Colonial Physician*, New York: Science History Publications, 1975. p. 1.
188 Abel, E. *Marihuana The First Twelve Thousand Years*, New York: Plenum, 1980. p. 79.
189 Grinspoon, L. *Marihuana Reconsidered*, Cambridge: Harvard University Press, 1971. p. 11.
190 Ibid. p. 11.
191 Ibid. p. 11.
192 Abel, E. *Marihuana The First Twelve Thousand Years*, New York: Plenum, 1980. p. 79.
193 Ibid. p. 79.
194 Ibid. p. 73.
195 Ibid. p. 73.
196 Simkins, F. *A History of the South*, New York: Alfred A. Knopf, 1956. p. 16.
197 Grinspoon, L. *Marihuana Reconsidered*, Cambridge: Harvard University Press, 1971. p. 12.
198 Sloman, L. *The History of Marihuana in America*, New York: Bobbs-Merrill, 1979. p. 21.
199 Grinspoon, L. *Marihuana Reconsidered*, Cambridge: Harvard University Press, 1971. p.12.
200 Wilson, J. *Appletons' Cyclopaedia of America*, New York: D. Appleton, 1889. p. 1.
201 Grinspoon, L. *Marihuana Reconsidered*, Cambridge: Harvard University Press, 1971. p. 12.
202 Abel, E. *Marihuana The First Twelve Thousand Years*, New York: Plenum, 1980. p. 119.
203 Ibid. p. 119.
204 Ibid. pp. 88-89.
205 Herer, J. *Hemp & The Marihuana Conspiracy*, Van Nuys: Queen of Clubs, 1993. p. 1.
206 Ibid. p. 5.
207 Bain, J. *Tobacco in Song and Story*, New York: New York Public Library, 1953. p. 126.
208 Abel, E. *Marihuana The First Twelve Thousand Years*, New York: Plenum, 1980. p. 89.
209 Ibid. p. 89.
210 Ibid. p. 90.
211 Ibid. p. 90.
212 Ibid. pp. 90-91.
213 Trowbridge, J. *The South*, Hartford, Connecticut: L. Stebbins, 1867. p. 189.
214 Abel, E. *Marihuana The First Twelve Thousand Years*, New York: Plenum, 1980. p. 90.
215 *World Book Encyclopedia, Volume 11 (J-K)*, Chicago: World Book Inc., 1995. p. 76.
216 Abel, E. *Marihuana The First Twelve Thousand Years*, New York: Plenum, 1980. p. 90.
217 Herer, J. *Hemp & The Marihuana Conspiracy*, Van Nuys: Queen of Clubs, 1993. p. 58.
218 Robinson, R. *The Great Book of Hemp*, Rochester: Park Street Press, 1996. Back Cover.
219 Ibid. p. 133.
220 Herer, J. *Hemp & The Marihuana Conspiracy*, Van Nuys: Queen of Clubs, 1993. p. 1.
221 Ibid. p. 1.
222 Abel, E. *Marihuana The First Twelve Thousand Years*, New York: Plenum, 1980. p. 90.
223 Ibid. p. 90.
224 Ibid. p. 90.
225 Ibid. p. 98.
226 Herer, J. *Hemp & The Marihuana Conspiracy*, Van Nuys: Queen of Clubs, 1993. p. 59.
227 Ibid. p. 59.
228 Herer, J. *Hemp & The Marihuana Conspiracy*, Van Nuys: Queen of Clubs, 1993. p. 60.
229 Steveacre, F. *Tea and Tea Drinking*, London: Sir Isaac Pitman & Sons, 1929. p. 1.
230 Ford, T. *The Apothecary in Eighteenth Century, Williamsburg*, Col: Williamsburg Pub., 1965. p. 3.
231 Abel, E. *Marihuana The First Twelve Thousand Years*, New York: Plenum, 1980. p. 98.

232 Ibid. p. 120.

233 Ibid. p. 120.

234 Ibid. p. 120.

235 Silverberg, R. *The Dawn of Medicine*, New York: G.P. Putnam's Sons, 1966. p. 49.

236 Abel, E. *Marihuana The First Twelve Thousand Years*, New York: Plenum, 1980. p. 120.

237 Herer, J. *Hemp & The Marihuana Conspiracy*, Van Nuys: Queen of Clubs, 1993. p. 36.

238 Abel, E. *Marihuana The First Twelve Thousand Years*, New York: Plenum, 1980. p. 120.

239 Ibid. p. 168.

240 Ibid. p. 168.

241 Ibid. p. 168.

242 Grinspoon, L. *Marihuana Reconsidered*, Cambridge: Harvard University Press, 1971.

243 Abel, E. *Marihuana The First Twelve Thousand Years*, New York: Plenum, 1980. p. 168.

244 Ibid. p. 169.

245 Ibid. p. 169.

246 Ibid. p. 169.

247 Herer, J. *Hemp & The Marihuana Conspiracy*, Van Nuys: Queen of Clubs, 1993. p. 9.

248 Ibid. p. 9.

249 Launert, E. *Perfumes and Pomanders*, Europe: Potterton, 1987. p. 173.

250 Robinson, R. *The Great Book Of Hemp*, Rochester: Park Street, 1996. pp. 47-48.

251 Abel, E. *Marihuana The First Twelve Thousand Years*, New York: Plenum, 1980. p. 169.

252 Ibid. p. 91.

253 Kane, H. *Plantation Parade*, New York: William Morrow & Co., 1945. p. 154.

254 Abel, E. *Marihuana The First Twelve Thousand Years*, New York: Plenum, 1980. p. 91.

255 Rouse, P. *Pioneers Life in Colonial Virginia*, New York: Hastings House, 1968. p. 198.

256 Grinspoon, L. *Marihuana Reconsidered*, Cambridge: Harvard University Press, 1971. p. 10.

257 Ibid. p. 10.

258 Sloman, L. *The History of Marihuana in America*, New York: Bobbs-Merrill, 1979. p. 22.

259 Ibid. p. 22.

260 Ibid. p. 22.

261 Ibid. p. 22.

262 American Spice Trade Association, *A Treasury of Spices*, New York: 1956. p. 21.

263 Bloomquist, E *Marijuana The Second Trip*, Beverly Hills: Glencoe, 1971. pp. 28-29.

264 Grinspoon, L. *Marihuana Reconsidered*, Cambridge: Harvard University Press, 1971. p. 13.

265 Montreal Museum of Fine Arts, *Exhibition of Kogo*, Montreal: 1978. p. 59.

266 Sloman, L. *The History of Marihuana in America*, New York: Bobbs-Merrill, 1979. p. 22.

267 Grinspoon, L. *Marihuana Reconsidered*, Cambridge: Harvard University Press, 1971. p. 218.

268 Ibid. p. 219.

269 Abel, E. *Marihuana The First Twelve Thousand Years*, New York: Plenum, 1980. p. 183.

270 Dare, M. *The 90's The Hemp Video*, Boulder: Instructional Tel. Foundation, 1990. Back Cover.

271 Locke, G. *The World Book*, Toronto: W.F. Quarrie & Co., 1923. p. 2195.

272 Abel, E. *Marihuana The First Twelve Thousand Years*, New York: Plenum, 1980. p. 183.

273 Locke, G. *The World Book*, Toronto: W.F. Quarrie & Co., 1923. p. 2195.

274 Ibid. p. 2195.

275 Dare, M. *The 90's The Hemp Video*, Boulder: Instructional Tel. Foundation, 1990. Back Cover.

276 Herer, J. *Hemp & The Marihuana Conspiracy*, Van Nuys: Queen of Clubs, 1993. p. 8.

277 The Rushlight Club. *Early Lighting*, Hartford: Finlay Bros., 1972. p. 17.

278 Stratton, D. *Candlesticks*, London: Pitman Publishing Ltd., 1976. p. 13.

279 Herer, J. *Hemp & The Marihuana Conspiracy*, Van Nuys: Queen of Clubs, 1993. p. 8.

280 Dare, M. *The 90's The Hemp Video*, Boulder: Instructional Tel. Foundation, 1990. Back Cover.

281 Grinspoon, L. *Marihuana Reconsidered*, Cambridge: Harvard University Press, 1971. p. 220.

282 Ibid. p. 220.

283 Ibid. p. 220.

284 Ibid. p. 220.

285 *The Imperial Encyclopaedic Dictionary*, London: Dictionary & Cyclopedia Co., 1901. p. 2165.

286 Grinspoon, L. *Marihuana Reconsidered*, Cambridge: Harvard University Press, 1971. p. 220.

287 Abel, E. *Marihuana The First Twelve Thousand Years*, New York: Plenum, 1980. p. 183.

288 Woodham-Smith, C. *Queen Victoria*, Great Britain: Hamish Hamilton, 1972. Front Cover.

289 Herer, J. *Hemp & The Marihuana Conspiracy*, Van Nuys: Queen of Clubs, 1993. p. 9.

290 Robinson, R. *The Great Book of Hemp*, Rochester: Park Street Press, 1996. p. 54.

291 Smith, M. *The Afternoon Tea Book*, New York: 1986. p. 20.

292 Herer, J. *Hemp & The Marihuana Conspiracy*, Van Nuys: Queen of Clubs, 1993. p. 2.

293 Robinson, R. *The Great Book of Hemp*, Rochester: Park Street Press, 1996. p. 54.

294 Montreal Museum of Fine Arts, *Boites a Encens Japonaises Redecouvertes*, Montreal: George Clemenceau Kogo Collection, 1978. p. 92.

295 Abel, E. *Marihuana The First Twelve Thousand Years*, New York: Plenum, 1980. p. 169.

296 Grinspoon, L. *Marihuana Reconsidered*, Cambridge: Harvard University Press, 1971. p. 221.

297 Ibid. p. 221.

298 Ibid. p. 221.

299 *Imperial Encyclopaedic Dictionary*, London: Dictionary & Cyclopedia Co., 1901. p. 2165.

300 Peat, Marwick, Mitchell and Co., *Marihuana A Study of State Policies and Penalties*, USA: Department of Justice, 1977. p. 61.

301 Rubin, V. *Cannabis and Culture*, Paris: Mouton Publishers, 1975. p. 46.

302 Fairholt, F. *Tobacco: Its History and Associations*, London: Chapman, 1859. p. 88.

303 Rubin, V. *Cannabis and Culture*, Paris: Mouton Publishers, 1975. p. 46.

304 Roth, J. *Old-Fashioned Candymaking*, Chicago: Henry Regnery Co., 1974. Cover.

305 Ruben, V. *Cannabis and Culture*, Paris: Mouton Publishers, 1975. pp. 46-47.

306 Ibid. p. 47.

307 Rosenthal, E. *Marihuana Growing Tips*, San Francisco: Quick American Publishing, 1986. p. 92.

308 Rubin, V. *Cannabis and Culture*, Paris: Mouton Publishers, 1975. p. 46.

309 Ibid. p. 46.

310 Ibid. p. 46.

311 Ibid. p. 46.

312 Ibid. p. 46.

313 Ibid. p. 46.

314 Fairholt, F. *Tobacco: Its History and Associations*, London: Chapman, 1859. p. 69.

315 Herer, J. *Hemp & The Marihuana Conspiracy*, Van Nuys: Queen of Clubs. 1993. p. 37.

316 United States Senate, *Marihuana and Health A Report to the Congress*, Washington, D.C.: U.S. Government Printing Office, 1971. pp. 53-54.

317 Merlin, J. *Man and Marihuana*, New Jersey: Fairleigh Dickinson University, 1972. p. 49.

318 Roth, J. *Old Fashioned Candy-Making*, Chicago: Henry Regnery Co., 1974. p. 64.

319 Herer, J. *Hemp & The Marihuana Conspiracy*, Van Nuys: Queen of Clubs, 1993. p. 64.

320 *Everyman's Encyclopaedia Volume 6*, London: J.M. Dent & Sons Ltd. 1967. p. 249.

321 Herer, J. *Hemp & The Marihuana Conspiracy*, Van Nuys: Queen of Clubs, 1993. p. 2.

322 Herer, J. *Hemp & The Marihuana Conspiracy*, Van Nuys: Queen of Clubs, 1993. p. 3.

323 Roulac, J. *Industrial Hemp*, Ojai, California: Hemptech, 1995. p. 8.

324 Merlin, M. *Man and Marijuana*, New Jersey: Fairleigh Dickinson University, 1972. p. 49.

325 Roulac, J. *Industrial Hemp*, Ojai, California: Hemptech, 1995. p. 9.

326 Grinspoon, L. *Marihuana Reconsidered*, Cambridge: Harvard University Press, 1971. p. 173.

327 Sloman, L. *The History of Marihuana in America*, New York: Bobbs-Merrill, 1979. p. 23.

328 Cannabis Canada, *Marijuana Is Medicine*, Vancouver, B.C.: Cannabis Canada, 1996. p. 2.

329 Grinspoon, L. *Marihuana Reconsidered*, Cambridge: Harvard University Press, 1971. p. 228.

330 Cheshire, F. *The Scientific Temperance Hand-Book*, London: Lorimer, 1891. p. 67.

331 Ibid. p. 66.

332 Ibid. p. 77.

333 Ibid. p. 77.

334 Ibid. p. 78.

335 Richmond, A. *Intemperance and Crime*, Cleveland: J. B. Savage, 1883. p. 44. (Chapter Six).

336 Ibid. p. 44. (Chapter Six).

337 Ibid. p. 45. (Chapter Six).

338 Ibid. p. 45. (Chapter Six).

339 Ibid. p. 46. (Chapter Six).

340 Daniels, W. *The Temperance Reform and Its Great Reformers*, New York: Nelson, 1878. p. 552.

341 Weatherall, M. *In Search Of A Cure*, New York: Oxford University Press, 1990. p. 146.

342 Daniels, W. *The Temperance Reform and Its Great Great Reformers*, New York: Nelson, 1878. p. 552.

343 Cheshire, F. *The Scientific Temperance Hand-Book*, London: Lorimer and Gillies, 1891. p. 71.

344 Daniels, W. *The Temperance Reform and Its Great Reformers*, New York: Nelson, 1878. p. 583.

345 Morrison, J. *Tempered By Rum*, Porters Lake, Nova Scotia: Pottersfield Press, 1988. p. 102.

346 Richmond, A. *Intemperance and Crime*, Cleveland: J.B. Savage, 1883. p. 231. (Postscript).

347 Ibid. pp. 104-105. (Chapter 14).

348 Furnas, J. *The life and Times of the Late Demon Rum*, New York: G.P. Putnam, 1965.

349 Asbury, H. *The Great Illusion An Informal History of Prohibition*, New York: Doubleday & Co., 1950. p. 9.

350 Richmond, A. *Intemperance and Crime*, Cleveland: J.B. Savage, 1883. p. 208. (Chapter 31).

351 Morrison, J. *Tempered By Rum*, Porters Lake, Nova Scotia: Pottersfield Press, 1988. p. 102.

352 Gough, J. *Platform Echoes: Living Truths For Head and Heart*, Hartford: Worthington, 1886. p. 85.

353 Richmond, A. *Intemperance and Crime*, Cleveland: J.B. Savage, 1883. p. 235. (Ch. 38).

354 Trotter, T. *Life Pictures From Rum's Gallery*, Toronto: Briggs, 1886. pp. 39-44. (Chapter 3).

355 Gough, J. *Platform Echoes: Living Truths For Head and Heart*, Hartford: Worthington, 1886. p. 431.

356 Richmond, A.B. *Intemperance and Crime*, Cleveland: J.B. Savage, 1883. pp. 168-169. (Chapter XXI).

357 Ibid. pp. 168-169. (Chapter XI).

358 Ibid. p. 71. (Chapter X).

359 Gough, J. *Platform Echoes: Living Truths For Head and Heart*, Hartford: Worthington, 1886. p. 402.

360 Richmond, A. *Intemperance and Crime*, Cleveland: J.B.Savage, 1883. p. 247. (Chapter XI).

361 Stamm, J. *The Ten Commandments in Recent Research*, London: SCM Press Ltd., 1962. p. 5.

362 Daiches, D. *Moses Man In the Wilderness*, London: Weidenfeld & Nicolson, 1975. Cover.

363 Gough, J. *Platform Echoes: Living Truths For Head and Heart*, Hartford: Worthington, 1886. p. 1.

364 Richmond, A. *Intemperance and Crime*, Cleveland: J.B. Savage, 1883. pp. 24-25. (Chapter IV).

365 Ibid. p. 196. (Chapter XXX).

366 Ibid. p. 196. (Chapter XXX).

367 Ibid. p. 197. (Chapter XXX).

368 Dickens, C. *Drinking With Dickens*, England: Mears, Caldwell, 1980. p. 38.

369 Richmond, A. *Intemperance and Crime*, Cleveland: J.B. Savage, 1883, p. 197. (Chapter XXX).

370 Ibid. p. 197. (Chapter XXX).

371 Ibid. p. 197. (Chapter XXX).

372 Ibid. p. 198. (Chapter XXX).

373 Cheshire, F. *The Scientific Temperance Hand-Book*, London: Lorimer & Gillies, 1981. p. 201.

374 Ibid. pp. 200-201.

375 Ibid. p. 201.

376 Richmond, A. *Intemperance and Crime*, Cleveland: J.B. Savage, 1883. p. 166. (Chapter XXV).

377 Ibid. p. 166. (Chapter XXV).

378 Cheshire, E. *The Scientific Temperance Hand-Book*, London: Lorimer, 1891. p. 158.

379 Gough, J. *Platform Echoes: Living Truths For Head and Heart*, Hartford: Worthington, 1886. p. 1.

380 Cheshire, E. *The Scientific Temperance Hand-Book*, London: Lorimer, 1891, p. 158.

381 Ibid. p. 158.

382 Ibid. p. 226.

383 Daniels, W. *The Intemperance Reform and Its Great Reformers*, New York: Nelson, 1878. p. 587.

384 Richmond, A. *Intemperance and Crime*, Cleveland: J.B. Savage, 1883. p. 170. (Chapter XXV).

385 Ibid. p. 52. (Chapter VI).

[386] Ibid. p. 52. (Chapter VI).

[387] Gough, J. *Platform Echoes: Living Truths For Head and Heart*, Hartford: Worthington, 1886. p. 1.

[388] Trotter, T. *Life Pictures From Rum's Gallery*, Toronto: Briggs, 1886. p. 341. (Chapter XXV).

[389] The Royal College of Physicians, *A Great and Growing Evil*, London: Tavistock, 1987. pp. 58-59.

[390] Willard, F.E. *How I Learned to Ride the Bicycle*, California: Fair Oaks Publishing, 1991. Cover.

[391] Trotter, T. *Life Pictures From Rum's Gallery*, Toronto: Briggs, 1886. pp. 344-347.

[392] Daniels, E. *The Intemperance Reform and Its Great Reformers*, New York: Nelson, 1878. pp. 339-340.

[393] Asbury, H. *The Great Illusion, An Informal History of Prohibition*, New York: Doubleday, 1950. p. 9.

[394] Adams, John. *The Founding Fathers*, New York: Harper & Row, 1961. p. 285.

[395] *Encyclopaedia Britannica, Volume 18*, Chicago: William Benton, 1972. p. 609.

[396] Adams, John. *The Founding Fathers*, New York: Harper & Row, 1961. p. 385.

[397] *Encyclopedia Americana International Edition Volume 22*, Connecticut: Grolier, 1982. p. 646.

[398] *Encyclopaedia Britannica Volume 18*, Chicago: William Benton, 1972. p. 609.

[399] Morrison, J. *Tempered By Rum*, Porters Lake, Nova Scotia: 1988. p. 152.

[400] Adams, John. *The Founding Fathers*, New York: Harper & Row, 1961. p. 68.

[401] *Encylcopaedia Britannica Volume 18*, Chicago: William Benton, 1972. p. 610.

[402] Randall, J. *Lincoln The President*, New York: Dodd, Mead & Co., 1956. p. 68.

[403] *The Book of Knowledge*, New York: Grolier, 1969. p. 125.

[404] Asbury, Herbert. *The Great Illusion, An Informal History of Prohibition*, New York: Doubleday, 1950. p. 94.

[405] Ibid. p. 99.

[406] *Encyclopaedia Britannica Volume 18*, Chicago: W. Benton, 1972. p. 610.

[407] Gough, J. *Platform Echoes: Living Truths For Head and Heart*, Hartford: Worthington, 1886. p. 1.

[408] Fredeman, W. *Pre-Raphaelitism*, Massachusetts: Harvard University Press, 1965. Insert.

[409] *Encyclopaedia Britannica Volume 18*, Chicago: W. Benton, 1972. p. 610.

[410] Ibid. p. 610.

[411] Ibid. p. 610.

[412] Cashman, S. *Prohibition The Lie of the Land*, London: Collier Macmillan, 1981. p. 29.

[413] Asbury, H. *The Great Illusion An Informal History of Prohibition*, New York: Doubleday, 1950. p. 135.

[414] Cashman, S. *Prohibition The Lie of the Land*, London: Collier Macmillan, 1981. p. 29.

[415] Everest, A. *Rum Across the Border*, New York: Syracuse University, 1978. Cover.

[416] Cashman, S. *Prohibition The Lie of the Land*, London: Collier Macmillan, 1981. p. 33.

[417] Ibid. pp. 30-31.

[418] Ibid. p. 32.

[419] Ibid. p. 29.

[420] Ibid. p. 262.

[421] Ibid. p. 262.

[422] Microsoft Internet Explorer. *The Complete History of Cannabis in Canada*, Microsoft Internet Explorer, Winnipeg: 1996. p. 1.

423 Ibid. p. 1.

424 Ibid. p. 2.

425 Ibid. p. 2.

426 Ibid. p. 2.

427 Ibid. p. 2.

428 Sherman, C. and Smith, A. *Highlights An Illustrated History of Cannabis*, Toronto: Ten Speed Press, 1999. p. 74.

429 Microsoft Internet Explorer, *The Complete History of Cannabis in Canada*, Microsoft Internet Explorer, Winnipeg: 1996. p. 2.

430 Ibid. p. 2.

431 Ibid. p. 2.

432 Ibid. p. 2.

433 Ibid. p. 2.

434 Cashman, S. *Prohibition The Lie of the Land*, London: Collier Macmillan, 1981. p. 262.

435 Fischer-Rizzi, S. *The Complete Incense Book*, New York: Sterling Publishing, 1998. p. 8.

436 Erickson, P. *Cannabis Criminals The Social Effects of Punishment on Drug Users*, Toronto: T.H. Best, 1980. p. 1.

437 Cashman, S. *Prohibition The Lie of the Land*, London: Collier Macmillan, 1981. p. 33.

438 Sloman, L. *The History of Marihuana in America*, New York: Bobbs-Merrill, 1979. p. 35.

439 Ibid. p. 36.

440 Ibid. p. 33.

441 Asbury, H. *The Great Illusion An Informal History of Prohibition*, New York: Doubleday, 1950. pp. 210-211.

442 Ibid. pp. 198-199.

443 *Encyclopedia Americana International Edition Volume 22*, Connecticut: Grolier, 1982. p. 648.

444 Asbury, H. *The Great Illusion An Informal History of Prohibition*, New York: Doubleday, 1950. p. 329.

445 *Encyclopaedia Britannica Volume 18*, Chicago: W. Benton, 1972. p. 611.

446 Sherman, C. and Smith, A. *Highlights An Illustrated History of Cannabis*, Toronto: Ten Speed Press, 1999. p. 104.

447 Robinson, R. *The Great Book of Hemp*, Rochester: Park Street Press, 1996. p. 151.

448 Ibid. p. 150.

449 Ibid. p. 150.

450 Ibid. p. 150.

451 Ibid. p. 152.

452 Ibid. p. 149.

453 Ibid. p. 149.

454 Ibid. p. 149.

455 Robinson, R. *The Great Book of Hemp*, Rochester: Park Street Press, 1996. p. 151.

456 *World Book*, Toronto: W.F. Quarrie & Co., 1923. p. 2262.

457 Ibid. p. 149.

458 Robinson, R. *The Great Book of Hemp*, Rochester: Park Street, 1996. p. 139.

459 Herer, J. *Hemp & The Marihuana Conspiracy*, Van Nuys: Queen of Clubs, 1993. p. 50.

460 Ibid. p. 45.

461 Robinson, R. *The Great Book of Hemp*, Rochester: Park Street, 1996. pp. 149-150.

462 Sloman, L. *The History of Marihuana in America*, New York: Bobbs-Merrill, 1979. p. 48.

463 Ibid. p. 113.

464 Herer, J. *Hemp & The Marihuana Conspiracy*, Van Nuys: Queen of Clubs, 1993. p. 28.

465 Clarke, R.C. *Hashish*, Los Angeles: Red Eye Press, 1998. p. CS6.

466 Robinson, R. *The Great Book of Hemp*, Rochester: Park Street Press, 1996. p. 14.

467 Herer, J. *Hemp & The Marihuana Conspiracy*, Van Nuys: Queen of Clubs, 1993. p. 28.

468 Ibid. p. 28.

469 Sloman, L. *The History of Marihuana in America*, New York: The Bobbs-Merrill Co., 1979. p. 80.

470 Fischer-Rizzi, S. *The Complete Incense Book*, New York: Sterling Publishing, 1998. p. 40.

471 Grinspoon, L. *Marihuana Reconsidered*, Cambridge: Harvard University Press, 1971. p. 226.

472 Herer, J. *Hemp & The Marihuana Conspiracy*, Van Nuys: Queen of Clubs, 1993. p. 10.

473 U.S. Senate, *Marihuana and Health A Report To The Congress*, Washington, D.C.: U.S. Government Printing Office, 1971. pp. 29 & 54.

474 Geller, A. & Boas, M. *The Drug Beat*, New York: Cowles, 1969. p. 82.

475 Robinson, R. *The Great Book of Hemp*, Rochester: Park Street, 1996. p. 47.

476 Herer, J. *Hemp & The Marihuana Conspiracy*, Van Nuys: Queen of Clubs, 1993. p. 63.

477 Robinson, R. *The Great Book Of Hemp*, Rochester: Park Street Press, 1996. p. 47.

478 Dunlop, R. *Doctors of the American Frontier*, New York: Doubleday, 1965. p. 133.

479 Dare, M. *The 90's Hemp Video*, Boulder: Instructional Tel. Foundation, 1990. Back Cover.

480 Finley, D. *A Standard of Excellence*, Washington, D.C.: Smithsonian Institution Press, 1973. p. 57.

481 Sloman, L. *The History of Marihuana in America*, New York: Bobbs-Merrill, 1979. p. 36.

482 Ibid. pp. 38-39.

483 Sherman, C. and Smith, A. *Highlights An Illustrated History of Cannabis*, Toronto: Ten Speed Press, 1999. p. 130.

484 Sloman, L. *The History of Marihuana in America*, New York: Bobbs-Merrill, 1979. pp. 44-45.

485 Geller, A. & Boas, M. *The Drug Beat*, Cowles, 1969. p. 120.

486 Corbett, J. *Turned On By God*, Richmond, Virginia: John Knox Press, 1971. p. 14.

487 Sloman, L. *The History of Marihuana in America*, New York: Bobbs-Merrill, 1979. p. 50.

488 Ibid. p. 76.

489 Herer, J. *Hemp & The Marihuana Conspiracy*, Van Nuys: Queen of Clubs, 1993. p. 29.

490 Himmelstein, J. *The Strange Career of Marihuana*, Connecticut: Greenwood Press, 1983. p. 91.

491 Ibid. p. 3.

492 Bloomquist, E. *Marijuana The Second Trip*, Beverly Hills: Glencoe, 1971. p. 253.

493 Rubin, V. *Cannabis and Culture*, Paris: Mouton Publishers, 1975. p. 498.

494 Bennett, C., Osburn, L.&J. *Green Gold The Tree of Life*, Cal.: Access Unlimited, 1995. p. 275.

495 Ibid. p. 274.

496 Ibid. p. 274.

497 Ibid. p. 274.

498 *Century Dictionary and Cyclopedia*, New York: Century Co., 1904. p. 2791.

499 Rosenthal, E. *Marijuana Growing Tips*, San Francisco: Quick American Publ., 1986. p. 93.

500 Sloman, L. *The History of Marihuana in America*, New York: Bobbs-Merrill, 1979. p. 122.

501 Grinspoon, L. *Marihuana Reconsidered*, Cambridge: Harvard University Press, 1971. p. 11.

502 Sloman, L. *The History of Marihuana in America*, New York: Bobbs-Merrill, 1979. p. 163.

503 Ibid. p. 153.

504 Ibid. p. 154.

505 Berry, R. & Boland, J. *The Economic Cost of Alcohol Abuse*, New York: Collier, 1977. p. 149.

506 *Encyclopedia Americana International Edition Volume 16*, Connecticut: Grolier, 1985. p. 668.

507 Bloomquist, E. *Marijuana The Second Trip*, Beverly Hills: Glencoe, 1971. pp. 230-236.

508 Fine, R. *Mary Jane Versus Pennsylvania*, New York: McCall, 1970. pp. 72-73.

509 Ibid. p. 73.

510 Government of Canada, *The Charter of Rights and Freedoms*, Ottawa: 1982. p. 15.

511 Government of Canada, *Canadian Charter of Rights and Freedoms*, Ottawa: 1982. Cover.

512 Sloman, L. *The History of Marihuana in America*, New York: Bobbs-Merrill, 1979. p. 162.

513 Barber, T. *LSD, Marihuana, Yoga, and Hypnosis in America*, Chicago: Aldine, 1970. p. 80.

514 Ibid. pp. 102-103.

515 Roulac, J. *Industrial Hemp*, Ojai, California: Hemptech, 1995. p. 14.

516 Herer, J. *Hemp & The Marihuana Conspiracy*, Van Nuys: Queen of Clubs, 1993. p. 47.

517 Ibid. p. 47.

518 Barber, T. *LSD, Marihuana, Yoga, and Hypnosis*, Chicago: Aldine, 1970. pp. 102-103.

519 U.S. Senate, *Marihuana and Health A Report to the Congress*, Washington, D.C.: U.S. Government Printing Office. 1971. p. 54.

520 Ibid. p. 54.

521 Sherman, C. and Smith, A. *Highlights An Illustrated History of Cannabis*, Toronto: Ten Speed Press, 1999. p. 13.

522 Barber, T. *LSD, Marihuana, Yoga and Hypnosis*, Chicago: Aldine, 1970. p. 98.

523 Fine, R. *Mary Jane Versus Pennsylvania*, New York: McCall, 1970. p. 52.

524 Ibid. pp. 52-53.

525 Herer, J. *Hemp & The Marihuana Conspiracy*, Van Nuys: Queen of Clubs, 1993. p. 71.

526 Himmelstein, J. *The Strange Career of Marihuana*, Westport: Greenwood, 1983. p. 90.

527 Sloman, L. *The History of Marihuana in America*, New York: Bobbs-Merrill, 1979. pp. 133-134.

528 Ibid. p. 187.

529 Clarke, R.C. *Hashish!* Los Angeles: Red Eye Press, 1998. p. 172.

530 Sloman, L. *The History of Marihuana in America*, New York: Bobbs-Merrill, 1979. p. 188.

531 *New Webster Encyclopedic Dictionary*, Chicago: Consolidated, 1971. p. 556.

532 Sloman, L. *The History Of Marihuana in America*, New York: Bobbs-Merrill, 1979. p. 189.

533 Ibid. p. 193.

534 Ibid. p. 228.

535 Schachner, N. *Thomas Jefferson*, London: Thomas Yoseloff Inc., 1957. Cover.

536 Robinson, R. *The Great Book of Hemp*, Rochester: Park Street Press, 1996. p. 188.

537 Geller, A. & Boas, M. *The Drug Best*, New York: Cowles, 1969. pp. 82-83.

538 Ibid. p. 121.

539 Ibid. p. 121.

540 Ibid. p. 121.

541 *World Book Encyclopedia Volume 5(D)*, London: World Book, 1994. p. 87.

542 Grinspoon, L. *Marihuana Reconsidered*, Cambridge: Harvard University, 1971. p. 229.

543 Rubin, Vera. *Cannabis and Culture*, Paris: Mouton Publishers, 1975. p. 70.

544 Ibid. p. 71.

545 Ibid. p. 71.

546 Bloomquist, E. *Marijuana The Second Trip*, Beverly Hills: Glencoe, 1971. p. 280.

547 Himmelstein, J.L. *The Strange Career of Marijuana*, Westport: Greenwood, 1983. pp. 90-91.

548 Louria, D. *The Drug Scene*, New York: MacGraw-Hill, 1968. p. 98.

549 Barber, T. *LSD, Marihuana, Yoga, and Hypnosis*, Chicago: Aldine, 1970. p. 100.

550 Sloman, L. *The History of Marihuana in America*, New York: Bobbs-Merrill, 1979. p. 163.

551 Clarke, R.C. *Hashish*, Los Angeles: Red Eye Press, 1998. p. CS7.

552 Sloman, L. *The History of Marihuana in America*, New York: Bobbs-Merrill, 1979. p. 164.

553 Tucker Fettner, A. *Potpourri, Incence*, New York: Workman, 1977. p. 106.

554 Barber, T. *LSD, Marihuana, Yoga, and Hypnosis*, Chicago: Aldine, 1970. p. 99.

555 Ibid. p. 99.

556 Herer, J. *Hemp & The Marihuana Conspiracy*, Van Nuys: Queen of Clubs, 1993. p. 34.

557 Flowers, T. *Marijuana Herbal Cookbook*, Berkeley: Rosetta Books, 1995. p. 80.

558 Herer, J. *Hemp & The Marihuana Conspiracy*, Van Nuys: Queen of Clubs, 1993. p. 38.

559 *Chambers's Encyclopaedia Volume V*, London: J.B. Lippincott, 1924, p. 639.

560 Geller, A. & Boas, M. *The Drug Beat*, New York: Cowles, 1969. p. 121.

561 Ibid. p. 31.

562 Ibid. p. 31.

563 Ibid. p. 31.

564 Fine, R. *Mary Jane Versus Pennsylvania*, New York: McCall, 1970. p. 54.

565 Ibid. p. 54.

566 Ibid. p. 59.

567 U.S. Senate. *Marihuana and Health A Report to the Congress*, Washington, D.C.: U.S. Government Printing Office, 1971. p. 92.

568 Government of Canada, *Canadian Charter of Rights and Freedoms*, Ottawa: 1982. p.1.

569 Robinson, R. *The Great Book of Hemp*, Rochester: Park Street Press, 1996. p. 189.

570 Bennett, C., Osburn, L.&J. *Green Gold The Tree of Life*, Cal.: Access Unlimited, 1995. p. 300.

571 Corbett, J. *Turned On By God*, Richmond: John Knox Press, 1971. p. 13.

572 Fine, R. *Mary Jane Versus Pennsylvania*, New York: McCall, 1970. p. 36.

573 Ibid. pp. 39-40.

574 Bennett, C., Osburn, L.&J. *Green Gold The Tree of Life*, Cal.: Access Unlimited, 1995. p. 44.

575 Ibid. p. 40.

576 *World Book Encyclopedia Volume 21*, Chicago: World Book, 1990. pp. 101-102.

577 Boswell, R. *Emily Murphy*, Calgary Herald, Calgary, Alta.: Mar. 7, 2004. p. A.5.

578 Boswell, R. *She Started the War on Weed*, Ottawa Citizen, Ottawa, Ont: Mar. 8, 2004. p. A4.

579 Moore, C. *Pot Should Be Legal*, Daily News, Halifax, N.S.: Sept. 20, 2002. p. 19.

580 Berry, R. & Boland, J. *The Economic Cost of Alcohol Abuse*, New York: Collier, 1977. p. 122.

581 Herer, J. *Hemp & The Marihuana Conspiracy*, Van Nuys: Queen of Clubs, 1993. p. 35.

582 Berry, R. & Boland, J. *The Economic Cost of Alcohol Abuse*, New York: Collier, 1977. pp. 130-131.

583 WHO Scientific Group, *The Use of Cannabis*, Geneva: World Health Organization, 1971. p. 17.

584 Boswell, R. *How the Marijuana Manace Began*, Times-Colonist, Victoria, B,C,: Mar. 14, 2004.

585 Bello, J. *The Physical, Psychological, Spiritual Benefits of Marijuana*, Penn: Lifeser., 1992. p. 43.

586 Chamber's *Encyclopaedia Volume V*, London: J.B. Lippincott, 1924. p. 639.

587 U.S. Senate, *Marihuana and Health*, Washington, D.C.: Government Printing Office, 1971. p. 54.

588 Herer, J. *Hemp and the Marihuana Conspiracy*, Van Nuys: Queen of Clubs, 1993. p. 37-38.

589 Flowers, T. *Marijuana Herbal Cookbook*, Berkeley: Rosetta Books, 1995. p. 79.

590 Herer, J. *Hemp & The Marihuana Conspiracy*, Van Nuys: Queen of Clubs, 1993. p. 219.

591 Ibid. p. 203.

592 U.S. Senate. *Marihuana and Health*, Washington, D.C.: Government Printing Office, 1971. p. 54.

593 Connell, P. & Dorn, N. *Cannabis and Man*, New York: Churchill Livingstone, 1975. p. 224.

594 Peat, Marwick, Mitchell & Co. *Marijuana A Study of State Policies & Penalties*, Washington: U.S. Dept. of Justice, 1977. p. 3

595 Sherman, C. and Smith, A. *An Illustrated History of Cannabis*, Toronto: Ten Speed Press, 1999. p. 113.

596 Herer, J. *Hemp & The Marihuana Conspiracy*, Van Nuys: Queen of Clubs, 1993. p. 38.

597 Flowers, T. *Marijuana Herbal Cookbook*, Berkeley, Rosetta Books, 1995. p. 81.

598 Robinson, R. *The Great book of Hemp*, Rochester: Park Street Press, 1996. p. 54.

599 Fischer-Rizzi, S. *The Complete Incense Book*, New York: Sterling Publishing, 1998. p. 10.

600 Flowers, T. *Marijuana Herbal Cookbook*, Berkeley, Rosetta Books, 1995. p. 81.

601 Herer, J. *Hemp & The Marihuana Conspiracy*, Van Nuys: Queen of Clubs, 1993. p. 39.

602 Rubin, V. *Cannabis and Culture*, Paris: Mouton Publishers, 1975. p. 72.

603 Ibid. p. 72.

604 Ibid. p. 72.

605 Ibid. pp. 72-73.

606 Herer, J. *Hemp & The Marihuana Conspiracy*, Van Nuys: Queen of Clubs, 1993. p. 37.

607 Sloman, L. *The History of Marihuana in America*, New York: Bobbs-Merrill, 1979. p. 311.

608 Erickson, P. *Cannabis Criminals*, Toronto: T.H. Best, 1980. p. 31.

609 *New International Encyclopaedia Volume XI*, New York: Dodd Mead, 1922. Insert.

610 Burne-Jones, E. *The Beginning of the World*, London: Longmans, Green, 1902. pp. 12-19.

611 Fine, R. *Mary Jane Versus Pennsylvania*, New York: McCall, 1970. pp. 35-70.

612 Erickson, P. *Cannabis Criminals*, Toronto: T.H. Best, 1980. p. 4.

613 Himmelstein, J. *The Strange Career of Marijuana*, Westport: Greenwood Press, 1983. p. 102.

614 Ibid. pp. 104-105.

615 Drey, R. *Apothecary Jars*, London: Faber & Faber, 1978. p. 127.

616 Himmelstein, J. *The Strange Career of Marijuana*, Westport: Greenwood Press, 1983. p. 104.

617 Brune-Jones, E. *The Beginning Of The World*, London: Longmans Green, 1902. pp. 12-19.

618 Fine, R. *Mary Jane Versus Pennsylvania*, New York: McCall, 1970. p. 9.

619 Ibid. p. 9.

[620] Ibid. pp. 9-10.

[621] Mazlish, B. *James and John Stuart Mill*, New York: Basic Books Inc., 1975. p. 152.

[622] Ibid. pp. 16-17.

[623] *The Moral Evolution Issue, Potshot #15*, Vancouver, B.C.: Cannabis Cannada, 2000. p. 28.

[624] Fine, R. *Mary Jane Versus Pennsylvania*, New York: McCall, 1970. p. 15.

[625] Ibid. p. 72.

[626] Ibid. p. 73.

[627] Ibid. p. 77.

[628] Bell, M. *The Politics of Pot*, Vancouver, B.C.: Vancouver Echo, Mar. 6. 1996. p. 3.

[629] Ibid. pp. 3-4.

[630] Sloman, L. *The History of Marihuana in America*, New York: Bobbs-Merrill, 1979. p. 245.

[631] *New Webster Encyclopedic Dictionary*, Chicago: Consolidated, 1971. p. 184.

[632] Burne Jones, E. *The Beginning Of The World*, London: Longmans Green, 1902. pp. 12 & 19.

[633] *World Book Encyclopedia Volume 19 (T)*, Toronto: World Book, 1992. p. 463.

[634] Ibid. p. 463.

[635] Government of Canada, *Canadian Charter of Rights and Freedoms*, Ottawa, 1982. p. 1.

[636] Ibid. p. 1.

[637] Ibid. p. 1.

[638] Ibid. p. 1.

[639] Ibid. p. 1.

[640] Herer, J. *Hemp & The Marihuana Conspiracy*, Van Nuys: Queen of Clubs, 1993. p. 87.

[641] Ibid. p. 41.

[642] Robinson, R. *The Great Book of Hemp*, Rochester: Park Street Press, 1996. p. 47.

[643] *World Book Encyclopedia Volume 19 (T)*, Chicago: World Book Inc., 2007. p. 463.

[644] Government of Canada, *Canadian Charter of Rights and Freedoms*, Ottawa: 1982. p. 1.

[645] Herer, J. *Hemp and the Marihuana Conspiracy*, Van Nuys: Queen of Clubs, 1993. p. 79.

[646] Bell, M. *The Politics of Pot*, Vancouver, B.C.: Vancouver Echo, Mar. 6. 1996. p. 4.

[647] Ibid. p. 4.

[648] Ibid. p. 4.

[649] *High Times*, New York: Trans-High Co., Feb. 1996. p. 50.

[650] Senate of Canada, *Public Hearings For Bill C-8 Transcripts*, Ottawa: 1996, p. 0950-2.

[651] Herer, J. *Hemp & The Marihuana Conspiracy*, Van Nuys: Queen of Clubs, 1993. p. 39.

[652] Ibid. p. 39.

[653] Ibid. p. 40.

[654] Ibid. p. 37.

[655] Ibid. p. 82.

[656] *Hemp Magazine*, Houston, Texas: March 1997. p. 18.

[657] Dare, M. *The 90s Hemp Video*, Boulder: Instructional Tel. Found. 1990. Cover.

[658] Gorman, P. *Marijuana and AIDS*, New York: Trans-High Co., 1994.p. 26.

[659] Ibid. pp. 27-28.

[660] Clarkes, L. *Just Say Grow*, Vancouver: Hemp B.C., 1996. Cover.

[661] Gorman, P. *Marijuana and AIDS*, New York: Trans-High Co., 1994. pp. 28 & 42.

[662] Herer, J. *Hemp & The Marihuana Conspiracy*, Van Nuys: Queen of Clubs, 1993. p. 9.

[663] Flowers, T. *Marijuana Herbal Cookbook*, Berkeley: Rosetta Books, 1995. p. 5.

[664] Herer, J. *Hemp & The Marihuana Conspiracy*, Van Nuys: Queen of Clubs, 1993. p. 43.

[665] Ibid. p. 43.

666 Ibid. p. 42.

667 Chapman, P. *What And How It Helps*, Vancouver, B.C.: The Province, Oct. 4, 1995. p. A5.

668 Flowers, T. *Marijuana Herbal Cookbook*, Berkeley: Rosetta Books, 1995. p. 6.

669 Ibid. p. 76.

670 Ibid. p. 82.

671 *High Times*, New York: Trans-High Co., Feb. 1996. p. 46.

672 Flowers, T. *Marijuana Herbal Cookbook*, Berkeley: Rosetta Books, 1995. pp. 70-71.

673 Ibid. p. 11.

674 Ibid. p. 2.

675 Herer, J. *Hemp & The Marihuana Conspiracy*, Van Nuys: Queen of Clubs, 1993. p. 35.

676 Robinson, R. *The Great Book of Hemp*, Rochester: Park Street Press, 1996. p. 53.

677 Herer, J. *Hemp & The Marihuana Conspiracy*, Van Nuys: Queen of Clubs, 1993. p. 35.

678 Ibid. p. 39.

679 Ibid. p. 41.

680 Ibid. p. 2.

681 *High Times*, New York: Trans-High Co., Feb. 1996. Cover.

682 Robinson, R. *The Great Book of Hemp*, Rochester: Park Street Press, 1995. p. 51.

683 Herer, J. *Hemp & The Marihuana Conspiracy*, Van Nuys: Queen of Clubs, 1993. p. 84.

684 Roulac, J. *Industrial Hemp*, Ojai: Hemptech, 1995. p. 18.

685 Herer, J. *Hemp & The Marihuana Conspiracy*, Van Nuys: Queen of Clubs, 1993. p. 44.

686 Sherman, C. and Smith, A. *Highlights An Illustrated History of Cannabis*, Toronto: Ten Speed Press, 1999. p. 22.

687 Herer, J. *Hemp & The Marihuana Conspiracy*, Van Nuys: Queen of Clubs, 1993. p. 10.

688 Romi, A. *Marijuana Law Ignores Benefits*, Regina, Sask.: Leader Post, June 26, 2003. p. B12.

689 Ibid. p. B12.

690 *Hemp News Magazine*, Houston, Texas: Feb. 1997. p. 14.

691 Barth, R. *Hemp's Energy Promise*, Nelson, B.C.: Nelson Daily News, Jul. 11, 2005. p. 4.

692 Ibid. p. 4.

693 Bell, M. *The Politics of Pot*, Vancouver: Vancouver Echo, Mar. 6, 1996. p. 4.

694 Launert, E. *Perfume and Pomanders*, Europe: Potterton Books, 1987. p. 116.

695 Wood, D. *War Without Winners*, Vancouver: Georgia Straight, 1995. pp. 11 & 13.

696 Ibid. p. 15.

697 Middleton, G. *Quit Filing Drug Possession Charges*, Vancouver: The Province, May 17, 1995. p. A5.

698 *Vancouver Sun*, Vancouver: July 20, 1995. p. B4.

699 Larsen, D. *Bill C-8: The Controlled Drugs and Substances Act --- Before the Senate*, Vancouver: Cannabis Canada, June, 1996. p. 18.

700 Ibid. p. 18.

701 Ibid. p. 18.

702 *High Times*, New York: Trans-High, Apr. 1997. p. 44.

703 Sherman, C. and Smith, A. *Highlights An Illustrated History of Cannabis*, Toronto: Ten Speed Press, 1999. p. 113.

704 *High Times*, New York: Trans-High Co., 1997. p. 46.

705 Ibid. p. 48.

706 *High Times*, New York: Tans-High, Nov. 1996. p. 39.

707 *High Times*, New York: Trans-High, Apr. 1997. p. 65.

708 *Hemp Magazine*, Houston, Texas: Feb. 1997. p. 8.

709 Ibid. p. 8.

710 Ibid. p. 18.

711 Sherman, C. and Smith, A. *Highlights An Illustrated History of Cannabis*, Toronto: Ten Speed Press, 1999. p. 9.

712 Clarke, R.C. *Hashish*, Los Angeles: Red Eye Press, 1998. p. 9.

713 Hrynyshyn, J. *Vancouver Sun*, Vancouver: May 28, 1986. p. A6.

714 Ibid. p. A6.

715 Ibid. p. A6.

716 Ibid. p. A6.

717 Vienneau, D. *Cultivating, Selling Hemp Stock Now Legal*, Toronto: The Toronto Star, June 21, 1996. p. A13.

718 Ibid. p. A13.

719 Hamilton, G. *Farmers Ready to Reap Rewards From Hemp Crops*, Vancouver: Vancouver Sun, Feb. 19, 1998. p. D20.

720 Sherman, C. and Smith, A. *Highlights An Illustrated History of Cannabis*, Toronto: Ten Speed Press, 1998. p. 8.

721 Government of Canada, *Canadian Charter of Rights and Freedoms*, Ottawa: 1982. p. 1.

722 Hamilton, S. *B.C. Pushing For More Hemp Farms*, Vancouver: The Province, June 15, 1997. p. A19.

723 Hamilton, S. *B.C. Co-op Told It Can Grow Hemp*, Vancouver: The Province, June 12, 1997. p. A9.

724 Leahy, S. *Industry Rediscovered*, Toronto: The Toronto Star, Sept. 14, 1996. p. C6.

725 Sherman, C. and Smith, A. *Highlights An Illustrated History of Cannabis*, Toronto: Ten Speed Press, 1998, p. 131.

726 Ravensbergen, J. *Industrial Hemp On the Rise Again*, Calgary: The Calgary Herald, Dec. 30, 1996.

727 Leahy, S. *Industry Rediscovered*, Toronto: The Toronto Star, Sept. 14, 1996. p. C6.

728 Ibid. p. C6.

729 Hamilton, S. *B.C. Pushing For More Hemp Farms*, Vancouver: The Province, June 15, 1997. p. A19.

730 Hamilton, S. *B.C. Co-op Told It Can Grow Hemp*, Vancouver: The Province, June 12, 1997. p. A9.

731 Clarke, R.C. *Hashish*, Los Angeles: Red Eye Press, 1998. p. xxiii.

732 Canadian Press, *Health Minister Approves Cultivation of Hemp*, Vancouver: Vancouver Sun, Feb. 27, 1998. p. A12.

733 Hamilton, G. *Farmers Ready To Reap Rewards From Hemp Crops*, Vancouver: Vancouver Sun, Feb. 19, 1998. p. D20.

734 Ibid. p. D20.

735 Ibid. p. D20.

736 Ibid. p. D20.

737 Sherman, C. and Smith, A. *Highlights An Illustrated History of Cannabis*, Toronto: Ten Speed Press, 1998. p. 15.

738 Canadian Press, *Health Minister Unveils Rules For Growing Hemp*, Tillsonburg: Calgary Herald, March 14, 1998. p. A16.

739 Ibid. p. A16.

740 Ibid. p. A16.

[741] MacLean, M. *Farmers Allowed To Grow 10 Acres But Caution Urged*, Calgary, Alta: Calgary Herald, April 20, 1998. p. C1.

[742] *High Hopes For Success*, Black Creek, The Province, July 6, 1998. p. A8.

[743] Ibid. p. A8.

[744] Hall, J. *The Miracle Crop*, Toronto: Toronto Star, May 25, 1998. pp. D1 & D3.

[745] Darroch, W. *Cannabis Helps Epileptics, Eases Pain, MD Tells Court*, Toronto: Toronto Star, Oct. 22, 1997. p. A33.

[746] Ibid. p. A33.

[747] Ibid. p. A33.

[748] Kines, L. *Marijuana Law Unconstitutional*, Vancouver, B.C.: Vancouver Sun, Aug. 1, 2000. pp. A1 & A2.

[749] *Grass Law Challenged*, Prince Rupert, B.C.: Daily News, Mar. 16, 2001. p. 5.

[750] Kines, L. *Marijuana Law Unconstitutional*, Vancouver, B.C.: Vancouver Sun, Aug. 1, 2000. p. A1.

[751] Tibbetts, J. *Anti-Marijuana Law Violates Rights of the Sick, Judge Rules*, Ottawa, Ont.: The Ottawa Citizen, Aug. 1, 2000. p. A3.

[752] Boswell, R. *Edmonton Crusader Blamed For Pot Prohibition*, Edmonton, Alta.: Edmonton Journal, Mar. 5, 2004. p. A1.

[753] Powell, B. & Cockburn, N. *Prosecutors Uncertain How They Will React*, Toronto, Ont.: Toronto Star, Oct. 8, 2003. p. A22.

[754] Boswell, R. *Edmonton Crusader Blamed For Pot Prohibition*, Edmonton, Alta: Edmonton Journal, Mar. 5, 2004. p. A1.

[755] Mayer, C. *DEA Puts The Bite on Hemp Chips*, Montreal, Que.: The Gazette, Jan. 15, 2002. p. B1.

[756] Boswell, R. *Edmonton Crusader Blamed For Pot Prohibition*, Edmonton, Alta.: Edmonton Journal, Mar. 5, 2004. p. A1.

[757] *Marijuana Activist brings Pro-Pot Arguement to Canada's Supreme Court*, Fort St. John, B.C.: Alaska Highway News, May 8, 2003.

[758] Powell, B. & Cockburn, N. *Prosecutors Uncertain How They Will React*, Toronto, Ont.: Toronto Star, Oct. 8, 2003, p. A22.

[759] Ibid. p. A22.

[760] Powell, B. & Cockburn, N. *Prosecutors Uncertain How They will React*, Toronto, Ont: Toronto Star, Oct. 8, 2003, p. A22.

[761] Bailey, S. *Possession of Small Amounts of Pot Remains Illegal*, Whitehorse, Y.T.: Whitehorse Star, Dec. 23, 2003. p. 8.

[762] Brown, J. *Top Court to Rule on Pot Law*, Windsor, Ont: Windsor Star, Dec. 18, 2003. p. B1.

[763] Pearson, C. *Activist Says Pot Sales Were Legal*, Windsor, Ont.: Windsor Star, Aug. 4, 2004. p. A1.

[764] Boswelll, R. *Edmonton Crusader Blamed for Pot Prohibition*, Edmonton, Alta.: Edmonton Journal, Mar. 5, 2004. p. A1.

[765] Barth, R. *Marc Emery and Cross-Border Seed Sales*, New Westminster, B.C.: Coquitlam Now, Aug. 6, 2005. p. 15.

[766] Ibid. p. 15.

[767] *The Alarming Global Reach of U.S. Law*, Sudbury, Ont.: Sudbury Star, Aug. 18, 2005. p. A10.

[768] Fairholt, F. *Tobacco: Its History and Associations*, London: Chapman, 1859. p. 181.

769 Ibid. p. 11.

770 *High Times*. New York: Trans-High Co., Feb. 1996. p. 45.

771 Herer, J. *Hemp & The Marihuana Conspiracy*, Van Nuys: Queen of Clubs, 1993. p. 43.

772 *High Times*, New York: Trans-High Co., Feb. 1996. p. 45.

773 Fischer-Rizzi, S. *The Complete Incense Book*, New York: Sterling Publishing, 1998. p. 136.

774 *High Times*. New York: Trans-High Co., 1995. Insert.

775 Gordon, S. *Marijuana: The Debate*, Montreal, Que: The Gazette, Oct. 24, 2002. p. A1.

776 Sherman, C. & Smith, A. *Highlights An Illustrated History of Cannabis*, Toronto: Ten Speed Press, 1999. p. 33.

777 Ibid. p. 131.

778 Boswell, R. *Edmonton Crusader Blamed For Pot Prohibition*, Edmonton, Alta.: Edmonton Journal, Mar. 5, 2004. p. A1.

779 Ibid. p. A1.

780 Richmond, A. *Intemperance and Crime*, Cleveland: J.B. Savage, 1883. pp. 50-51.

781 *New Educator Encyclopedia Volume 3*, Toronto: General Press, 1956. p. 926.

782 Randall, J. *Lincoln The President*, New York: Dodd, Mead, 1956. p. 68.

783 *New Educator Encyclopedia, Volume 5*, Toronto: General Press, 1956. p. 1514A.

784 Fischer-Rizzi, S. *The Complete Incense Book*, New York: Sterling Publishing, 1998. p. 10.

785 Tucker Fettner, A. *Potpourri, Incence*, New York: Workman, 1977. p. 106.

786 Sherman, C. and Smith, A. *Highlights An Illustrated History of Cannabis*, Toronto: Ten Speed Press; 1999. p. 113.

787 Schwarez, J. *Despite Decades of Propaganda, Cannabis is Proving Its Worth*, Montreal, Que.: The Gazette, Aug. 13, 2000. p. C4.

788 Ibid. p. C4.

789 Ibid. p. C4.

790 *High Times*, New York: Trans-High Co., May, 1997. pp. 20 & 22.

791 News Services, *Side-Effects Reviewed*, Ottawa, Ont.: The Province, Nov. 18, 1998. p. A24.

792 Lavergne, A. & Robinson, A. *Mellow Out On Pot Laws*, Chilliwack, B.C.: Chilliwack Times, Jan. 31, 2003. p. 8.

793 *Legalized Marijuana Would Help*, Nanaimo, B.C.: Nanaimo Daily News, Nov. 8, 2001. p. A8.

794 Barth, R. *Marc Emery and Cross-Border Seed Sales*, New Westminster, B.C.: Coquitlam Now, Aug. 6, 2005. p. 15.

795 Moore, C. *Pot Should Be Legal*, Halifax, N.S.: Daily News, Sept. 20, 2002. p. 19.

796 Sherman, O. *The Creation*, New York: Dial Books, 1990.

797 Harvey, W. *The Book*, Rogers, Arkansas: Mundus, 1930. p. 35.

798 Rhodehamel, J. *Foundations of Freedom*, Los Angeles: Constitutional Rights Foundation, 1991. p. 9.

799 Launert, E. *Perfume and Pomanders*, Europe: Potterton books, 1987. p. 116.

800 Fischer-Rizzi, S. *The Complete Incense Book*, New York: 1998. p. 150.